S0-AIV-926

Cooking for Health

Stress and Hypertension

Macrobiotic Food and Cooking Series

MACROBIOTIC FOOD AND COOKING SERIES

Cooking for Health

Stress and Hypertension

by Aveline Kushi

edited by Sarah Lapenta

foreword by Martha C. Cottrell M.D.

Japan Publications, Inc.

Tokyo · New York

© 1988 Japan Publications, Inc.

All rights reserved, including the right to reproduce this book or portions thereof in any form without the written permission of the publisher.

Note to the reader: Those with health problems are advised to seek the guidance of a qualified medical, or psychological professional in addition to that of a qualified macrobiotic counselor before implementing any of the dietary and other approaches presented in this book. It is essential that any reader who has any reason to suspect serious illness in themselves or their family members seek appropriate medical, nutritional, or psychological advice promptly. Neither this or any other health related book should be used as a substitute for qualified care or treatment.

Published by JAPAN PUBLICATIONS, INC., Tokyo and New York

Distributors:
UNITED STATES: *Kodansha International/USA, Ltd., through Harper & Row, Publishers, Inc., 599 Lexington Avenue, Suite 2300, New York, N. Y. 10022.* SOUTH AMERICA: *Harper & Row, Publishers, Inc., International Department.* CANADA: *Fitzhenry & Whiteside Ltd., 195 Allstate Parkway, Markham, Ontario, L3R 4T8.* MEXICO AND GENTRAL AMERICA: *HARLA S. A. ed C. V., Apartado 30–546, Mexico 4, D. F.* BRITISH ISLES: *Premier Book Marketing Ltd., 1 Gower Street, London WC1E 6HA.* EUROPEAN CONTINENT: *European Book Service PBD, Strijkviertel 63, 3454 PK De Meern, The Netherlands.* AUSTRALIA AND NEW ZEALAND: *Bookwise International, 1 Jeanes Street, Beverley, South Australia 5007.* THE FAR EAST AND JAPAN: *Japan Publications Trading Co., Ltd., 1-2-1, Sarugaku-cho, Chiyoda-ku, Tokyo 101.*

First edition: September 1988

LCCC No. 86–082769
ISBN 0–87040–679–5

Printed in U.S.A.

Foreword

In this book you will be presented with many facts about the nature of stress, hypertension, and other common stress-related conditions. You will be given scientific explanations concerning cause and development of these ailments, and you will be introduced to a highly dynamic perspective, the ancient principle of complementary opposites, yin and yang. As a coherent way of interpreting our world and ourselves, this unique perceptual tool continues to serve me well in both my personal and my professional life.

Through the illness of my mother, and later on, through my training and experience as a physician, I have come to see that *allopathic medicine* (drugs and surgery) and holistic medicine are complementary. Each has its own intrinsic merit; each offers valuable information and skills for the prevention and treatment of our major diseases. If only I had had this information to help my mother through her years of disability and suffering from both physical and mental degeneration. From my studies of macrobiotics, I am certain that her quality of life could have been greatly enhanced and that she could have lived a long and happy life.

My family history shows a considerable amount of heart disease, breast and colon cancer, allergies, and nervous disorders. I myself suffered early on from chronic sinusitis and digestive problems, and later on from bursitis, arthritis, arthritic scoriosis, and the effects of an extremely stressful lifestyle. Stress and anxiety pervaded my academic life in the predominantly male-oriented environment of medical school, and, subsequently, my professional life as a woman doctor. For many years, in an effort to "cope," I frequently ingested amphetamines, caffeine, sugar, junk foods, tabacco, and alcohol —until one day I decided to take charge of my life.

After practicing macrobiotics for seven years, and just turning sixty this past March, I find myself stronger and more vital in body, mind, and spirit than at age forty. After years of struggle, my personal and family life have begun to find a renewed harmony. For this I am very grateful to my teachers Michio and Aveline Kushi, Shizuko Yamamoto, Neil and Janet Stapleman, Bill Spear, Bill Tara, Murray Snyder, to my patients, and to my own commitment in applying this discipline on a daily basis.

As a physician, I deeply appreciate having this discipline to share with my patients. As a medical researcher, I appreciate being able to apply a growing body of scientific data to assess the validity of macrobiotic recommendations. All scientific studies are pointing toward

6

a diet high in complex carbohydrates and fiber, low in fat, and moderate in protein. The Standard Macrobiotic Diet is the only dietary pattern which attains this ideal while, at the same time, offering numerous benefits not considered in current guidelines issued by institutions such as the National Cancer Institute and the American Heart Association. For instance, by regularly including sea vegetables and organically grown whole grains and vegetables, the macrobiotic diet provides us with an abundance of valuable vitamins and minerals while minimizing our intake of chemical pollutants. This pattern of consumption not only promotes national health, but also promotes a more sustainable, ecological form of agriculture.

As we learn more about the interrelations of mind and body, about the role of stress in health and disease, the efficacy of macrobiotic principles becomes ever more clear. We now know, for instance, that emotional states can influence the immune system via the hormonal and nervous systems. In addition, nutritional scientists have discovered integral links between nutrition and brain chemistry, and between nutrition and the immune system. The delicate balance of health results from a complex interplay of emotions, nutrition, stress, and disease resistance. While modern psychological approaches to stress indeed have merit, their effects can be greatly enhanced by attending to diet and other practical aspects of health. Through its central emphasis on nutrition and ecology, macrobiotics provides the missing links to a comprehensive view of stress and the genesis of disease.

After seven years of practicing this way of life, I see endless possibilities unfolding for the regeneration of humanity. As we approach the end of the twentieth century, however, there is an urgent need for everyone to begin applying this important knowledge, the principles of balance and wholeness, to our daily way of life. We must be responsible to the conditions of deterioration within and around us, in our bodies and in the environment upon which our life ultimately depends.

Macrobiotics teaches us to respect our primordial bound to the natural world. As a way of self-healing, it affords us the experience of wholeness within ourselves and harmony with the rhythms of nature, including the changing seasons. It teaches us that self and society are not separate, that one individual's healing influences the health and well-being of society as a whole. Given the imminent social, economic, ecological, and political crises of our time, this process of healing can no longer be delayed. It is time to take our destiny into our own hands. I remain firmly committed to macrobiotics as a way to prevent disease and renew our health as individuals, as nations, and as one planetary community.

Martha C. Cottrell, M.D.
New York City, April 20, 1988

Preface ■■■■■■■■

About fifteen years ago, one of our friends studying in Boston was also a student at Harvard Medical School. He conducted a series of research projects with the macrobiotic community. He began visiting student houses in the Boston area with equipment to measure blood pressure. Many of our friends who were eating a macrobiotic diet and were active in the Boston community participated. The results of his efforts was tremendous. He checked the blood pressure of more than two hundred of our friends and found that they were substantially lower than that of the average American.

Our friend then conducted another study in which blood cholesterol levels were checked and then compared to a control population from the Framingham Heart Study. Our macrobiotic friends were found to have much lower cholesterol levels than the non-macrobiotic people. The researchers at Harvard and Framingham were very impressed by the extremely low cholesterol levels, which were among the lowest levels in any human population in the world.

The results helped to change the view of heart disease, so that by the mid-seventies, leading public health organizations, including the U.S. Senate Select Committee on Nutrition and Human Needs, the American Heart Association, and others began recommending a diet based around whole cereal grains, beans, and fresh vegetables as a way to prevent the buildup of cholesterol, high blood pressure, and other forms of heart disease.

The level of blood pressure is a common barometer of our response to stress. The interesting thing about the Harvard studies was that macrobiotic people were maintaining a relatively stress-free internal environment while living in the middle of one of the largest cities in North America. From this we can begin to see that stress is due largely to our diet and physical condition and not simply the result of our environment. Why is it, for example, that in a given environment one person will feel highly stressed while another remains more calm and relaxed? The difference must be due to each person's physical condition and make up, both of which are determined primarily by diet.

Over the years, I have met many people who were suffering from various types of stress, both physical and emotional, who were able to become more healthy and stress-free by changing their way of eating. Over the years, macrobiotic educational organizations including the East West Foundation and the Kushi Foundation have publicized case histories of people who were able to lower their blood pressure and cholesterol levels by following a balanced macrobiotic diet. For readers experiencing stress of any sort, the first step toward recovering a more natural balance is to begin eating a diet prepared in harmony with nature, using the best-quality ingredients. The recipes and information presented in this book and its companion volume in the *Macrobiotic Health and Education Series*, offer a practical way for everyone to recover from stress and to enjoy a harmonious, creative, and happy life.

I would like to thank all our friends who assisted in completing this book: I thank our associate Sarah Lapenta for compiling the recipes, menus, and related text, along with her husband Stephen. I thank our associates Ed and Wendy Esko for advice and inspiration, as well as our friends who assisted Michio Kushi in completing the companion volume, including Mark Mead, the editor of that volume. I also thank our friends who worked on the illustrations and artwork for the *Macrobiotic Food and Cooking Series:* Lillian Kushi, Jay Kelly, and Christian Gautier. I thank Mr. Iwao Yoshizaki and Mr. Yoshiro Fujiwara, respectively president and American representative of Japan Publications for their continuing inspiration. I would also like to thank Philip Jannetta and other members of the Japan Publications staff for their editorial work on this volume.

Aveline Kushi
Becket, Massachusetts
September, 1987

Contents

10

1. Understanding Macrobiotic Principles ━━━━━━━━

Among the many factors influencing our daily lives, none is more within our power to control than choosing which foods we eat. It then follows that a priority for health-conscious individuals will be learning how to choose and prepare delicious food that can maintain health, decrease sickness, and restore balance and harmony to their lifestyles. Macrobiotic cooking is the important first step in activating our intuition, allowing us to see, through practical experience, the means toward this end.

In the beginning, our practice of cooking relies on classes and cookbooks, each dish prepared precisely as the recipe calls for. With experience and improved judgment we begin to improvise and experiment, replacing measuring cups and clocks with our own sense of order and balance when preparing meals.

As our study and practice of cooking matures it is as if we are guided by an internal compass. The points on our compass are not north, south, east, or west, but are instead labeled by the unique philosophical basis of macrobiotics, the study of yin and yang. By learning to use this compass we can raise our practice of cooking to an art.

Yin and Yang: The Constitution of Nature━━━━

We live in a universe that is constantly in motion, always changing. From the movement of galaxies to electrons spinning around a nucleus all phenomena succumb to and are renewed by alternating currents of attraction and repulsion. In nature, summer changes to winter, day into night. Our hearts and lungs rhythmically contract and expand as our lives move from youth to old age. Often we experience love turning to hate then again to love. Joy and sorrow, wealth and poverty, and the rise and fall of civilizations complement each other in the same way as one tendency changes into its opposite and then returns to its original state.

These cycles of change occur throughout nature as the unifying principle that creates and maintains in balance our entire universe.

Throughout history many terms and symbols have been used to express the complementary and antagonistic relationships at play in the rhythm of the universe. In our study of macrobiotics the terms yin and yang embody the tendency to produce either expansion or contraction. *Yin* energy creates outward, centrifugal movement resulting in expansion, while *yang*, or inward, centripetal movement produces contraction.

Between the heavens and the planet earth these two forces are manifested as: 1) a downward, centripetal, or yang force generated

Attribute	Yin/Centrifugal (▽)	Yang/Centripetal(△)
Tendency	Expansion	Contraction
Function	Dispersion, decomposition	Assimilation, organization
Movement	More inactive, slower	More active, faster
Vibration	Shorter waves, high frequency	Longer waves, low frequency
Direction	Vertical, ascending	Horizontal, descending
Position	More outward and peripheral	More inward and central
Weight	Lighter	Heavier
Temperature	Colder	Hotter
Light	Darker	Lighter
Humidity	More wet	More dry
Density	Thinner	Thicker
Size	Larger	Smaller
Shape	More expanded, fragile	More contracted, harder
Length	Longer	Shorter
Texture	Softer	Harder
Atomic particle	Electron	Proton
Elements	N, O, K, P, Ca	H, C, Na, As, Mg
Environment	Vibration→Air→Water→	Earth
Climate	Tropical	Arctic
Biology	Vegetable	Animal
Sex	Female	Male
Organ structure	Hollow, expansive	Compact, condensed
Nerves	Orthosympathetic	Parasympathetic
Attitude	Gentle, negative	Active, positive
Work	Psychological & mental	Physical & social
Consciousness	More universal	More specific
Mental function	Dealing with the future	Dealing with the past
Culture	Spiritually oriented	Materially oriented
Color	Purple→Blue→Green→ Yellow→	Brown→Orange→Red
Season	Winter	Summer
Dimension	Space	Time
Taste	Hot→sour→sweet→	Salty→Bitter
Vitamins	C	K, D
Catalyst	Water	Fire

inward to the center of the earth by the sun, the stars, and far distant galaxies, and 2) an upward, centrifugal, or yin force generated outward due to the rotation of the earth. Universally referred to as the forces of Heaven and Earth, the attraction between these two forces creates and maintains biological life in an area encompassing the crust, waters, and atmosphere of our planet.

Within this biosphere and throughout the animal and vegetable kingdoms that exist there, balance between yin and yang is a natural process. Humanity, within the context of modern society, has lost sight of the laws of nature but has not been immune to their effects. The resulting rise in degenerative illness, war, and social problems attest to this. By adopting a simpler lifestyle and an appropriate diet we can rediscover our innate understanding of these natural laws.

The classifications of the antagonistic and complementary tendencies, yin and yang, on the opposite page show practical examples of these relative forces.

The key to understanding the influence of yin and yang lies in seeing the dominance of one or the other. Any phenomenon can be classified as either more yin or more yang by establishing its expansive or contractive tendency. Most importantly, while one always dominates, it is the combination of both forces that creates life. Just as our hearts beat, sending the pulse of life through our veins, yin and yang are the pulse of nature, alternating between expansion and contraction, action and rest, death and rebirth. As life ends with the cessation of our human pulse, so too would all phenomena cease to exist were it not for the constant pulsating of this natural rhythm.

Classifying Foods by Their Yin and Yang Tendencies

Food is our source of being. Through the vegetable kingdom all the basic forces of life are combined in a form that can be used by the human organism. Sunlight, soil, water, and air are taken in through the medium of the vegetable kingdom. To eat is to take in the whole environment.

As students of macrobiotic cooking our initial concern is understanding the influence of yin and yang on the foods we prepare. Toward this end the classification of foods into categories of yin and yang is essential for the development of a balanced diet. Different factors in the growth and structure of foods indicate whether the food is predominantly yin or yang. This is illustrated as followes:

Yin and Yang Influences on Plants

Yin Energy Creates:
Growth in a hot climate
Foods containing more water
Fruits and leaves
Growth high above the ground
An acid reaction in the body
Hot, aromatic foods

Yang Energy Creates:
Growth in a cold climate
Foods which are more dry
Stems, roots, and seeds
Growth below the ground
An alkaline reaction in the body
Salty, sour foods

To classify foods we must see the predominant factors, since all foods have yin and yang qualities. One of the most accurate methods of classification is to observe the cycle of growth in vegetables. During the winter, the climate is colder (yin); at this time of year energy descends into the root system. Leaves wither and die as the sap descends to the roots and the vitality of the plant becomes more condensed. Vegetables grown in the late autumn and winter are drier and more concentrated, and can be kept for a long time without spoiling. Some examples are carrots, parsnips, turnips, and cabbage. During the spring and early summer, energy ascends and new greens appear as the weather becomes hotter (yang). These vegetables are more yin in nature. Summer vegetables are more watery and perish quickly. They provide a cooling effect necessary in warm months while winter vegetables help preserve our inner warmth. In late summer, energy in the vegetable kingdom has reached its zenith and the fruits become ripe. They are very watery and sweet and develop higher above the ground.

This yearly cycle shows the alternation between predominating yin and yang energies as the seasons turn. This same cycle can be applied to the part of the world in which a food originates. Foods that originate in hot, tropical climates where the vegetation is lush and abundant, are more yin, while foods originating in more northern or colder climates are more yang.

Different vegetables that grow at the same time of the year are classified by their dominant direction of growth. The root system is governed by yang energy, the stem and leaves by yin energy.

In order to harmonize our diet with the rhythm of the seasons we select vegetables whose energy will balance the prevailing environmental conditions. When we plan menus in the warmer season of the year or in a warmer environment, it is appropriate to balance these yang factors with vegetables from the yin category. Conversely, when selecting vegetables in the colder season of the year or in colder regions, we can offset these yin environmental factors with a diet high in vegetables from the yang category.

Fig. 1 General Yin (▽) and Yang (△) Categorization of Foods

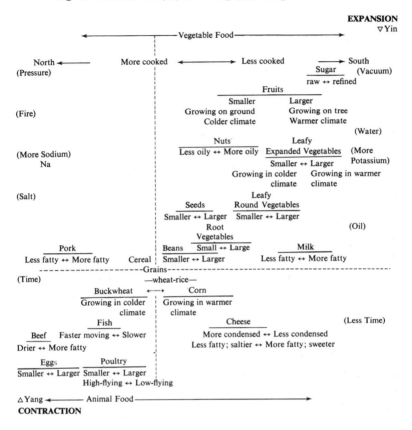

The above chart gives the general classification of food groups from yang to yin. However, more precise classification should be made upon examination of environmental conditions, nature and structure, chemical compounds, and effect upon our physical and mental conditions. Also, cooking can greatly change food qualities from yin to yang and yang to yin.

An understanding of the complementary and antagonistic relationship between the environment and the type of food produced, as expressed in the previous examples, plays an important part in creating a balanced diet. Other factors, such as our present condition and type of activity are also important. With time and practice, a natural sense of which foods are appropriate will evolve, so experiment freely and do not worry about making mistakes. By selecting from a wide variety of grains and vegetables, occasionally supplemented by a small amount of animal food, we can build a healthy foundation for whichever lifestyle we choose.

Food Spectrum from Yin to Yang ━━━━━━━━━━

We are now able to classify, from yang to yin or yin to yang, the entire scope of food. Generally speaking, animal food is extremely yang; fruits, dairy food, sugar, and spices are extremely yin; and grains, beans, and vegetables are more centered and fall in the middle of the spectrum. Within the category of extreme yang foods, we can classify from most yang to less yang the following: salt, eggs, meat, poultry, salty cheeses, and fish. In the category of extreme yin foods, from less yin to most yin, we find milk and other dairy products; tropical vegetables and fruits; coffee and tea; alcohol; spices; honey, sugar, soft drinks, and other sweetened foods; all food prepared with chemicals or artificial additives; marijuana, cocaine, and other drugs; and most medications. In the center of the spectrum, relative to each other, cereal grains are more yang, followed by beans, seeds, root vegetables, leafy round vegetables, leafy expanded vegetables, nuts, and fruits grown in a temperate climate.

Since we need to maintain a continually dynamic balance and harmony between yin and yang in order to adapt to our immediate environment, when we eat foods from one extreme, we are naturally attracted to the other. For example, a diet consisting of large quantities of meat, eggs, and other animal foods, which are very yang, requires a correspondingly large intake of foods in the extreme yin category such as tropical fruits, sugar, alcohol, spices, and, in some cases, drugs. However, a diet based on such extremes is very difficult to balance, often resulting in sickness caused by an excess of one of the two factors, or both.

The Importance of Cereal Grains ━━━━━━━━━━

Among our foods, the cereal grains are unique. As both seed and fruit, they combine the beginning and end of the growth cycle of plants and contain the most balanced proportion of carbohydrate, fat, protein, and mineral of any food. Among cereal grains, brown rice is the most balanced. Its size, shape, color, texture, and proportion of nutrients fall in the middle of the spectrum of cereal grains. As the most integrated of the cereals, brown rice is our evolutionary counterpart in the plant world.

It is for this evolutionary reason, and for the great ability of cereals to combine well with other vegetables and beans, that whole grains formed the principal food in most previous civilizations.

Throughout history all great civilizations cultivated one or more of the whole grains as their principal food. In the Orient rice has always been a staple; in northern Europe the staple food was *kasha*, or buckwheat; in various parts of central and western Europe it was wheat, barley, and oats; and in the Americas, whole corn was the basic food. The macrobiotic diet recommends brown rice as the principal grain. Now cultivated on every continent, brown rice may be considered humanity's universal staple.

Recently, the consumption of whole grains has fallen sharply. In its place animal-quality foods such as meat and dairy products, and refined carbohydrates such as sugar and refined flour have become the main food for most people. It is now widely recognized that this shift in diet has resulted in many of the major sicknesses that plague modern society.

As we stray further from a diet based on whole cereal grains, we begin to forfeit our ability to choose food wisely, instead succumbing to cravings and binges that lead to a chaotic lifestyle. By returning to a more centered diet we can regain our sense of direction and use food to create our lives, not destroy them.

Becoming a Macrobiotic Cook

To balance yin and yang we need to learn how to create, transform, and modify energy. Our body, our food, and our environment are changing forms and patterns of energy. Understanding the dynamics of change and applying it to all aspects of life to maximize our health and happiness is the goal of macrobiotics. To encourage this understanding in ourselves, our families, and our friends is the challenge confronting the macrobiotic cook.

The food we eat is a reflection of the cook's condition and judgment. The quality of food selected, the way it is cut, the length of cooking time, the amount of seasoning, how the meal is presented at the table, and its taste and flavor—all depend on the cook. Day in and day out the cook determines the health and well-being of the family. A cook whose own health is strong and whose judgment is sound creates food that is nourishing, satisfying, healing, and pleasing to behold. He or she is able to modify cooking according to the changing seasons or weather, the availability or scarcity of certain items, and the personal condition and needs of those for whom she cooks.

We begin simply with pressure-cooked brown rice, *miso* soup, and a few basic vegetable, bean, and sea vegetable dishes, while at the same time diminishing in volume the foods previously eaten. Gradually, condiments, pickles, and naturally sweetened desserts are introduced while frequently varying the combinations and styles of cooking so the food remains appealing and appetizing.

As we continue to prepare these foods, our own health and judgment will improve, our taste for natural food will deepen, and our ability to select the freshest items, prepare them properly, and arrange them in a beautiful meal will develop naturally.

While cookbooks can introduce you to macrobiotic food preparation, until you have actually tasted the foods and seen them prepared, you will not have a standard against which to measure your own cooking. In the beginning it is recommended that everyone study with an experienced macrobiotic cook. Only a few cooking lessons are needed to orient you in the right direction.

With experience you will eventually reach the point where you no longer need a cookbook or teacher but can use your own internal compass as a guide, and nature and the universe as primary instructors. By heeding their lessons and learning from your own mistakes all questions can be answered, all meals can be a part of the creation of life itself.

2. Understanding Stress and Hypertension

As modern society grows more complex, the challenge to our understanding and practice of a natural way of life becomes greater. The increasing disparity between a life in harmony with nature and one in synch with modern technology reveals a problem many people face and poses an inherent question to be answered by applying macrobiotic principles: How can we unify the two?

The pace of modern life differs from the less stressful and hurried style of life our parents and grandparents knew. There is less contact with nature. The earth, trees, and open spaces have been replaced with cement, glass, and the automobile. We shelter ourselves from the changing seasons with air conditioners, central heating, and vacations to different climates.

Most striking has been the deterioration of food quality and the effect it has had on personal health, and family and social relations.

Comparing Past and Present

Even as the trend towards industrialization prompted the move from country to city, our parents and grandparents were able to enjoy a primarily natural and unprocessed diet, based largely around complex carbohydrates in the form of whole grains, beans, and vegetables. In most cases this food was grown locally, available fresh and therefore free from chemical additives and preservatives. Cooking was one of the most important and ongoing activities in the home. As a result, the bonds joining family members and community remained strong.

Lacking many of the modern conveniences available today, daily tasks required more physical activity which facilitated the discharge of excess calories and other factors in the diet. Preparing meals, cleaning, heating the home, and similar chores bridged the gap between work and play when shared by friends and family members. Without the distraction of television there was ample time for quiet reflection. The natural cycle of retiring early and rising with the sun was enjoyed without the aid of an alarm clock.

These combined factors: a diet consisting of natural, regional food from complex-carbohydrate sources, prepared for and shared by the entire family; together with regular activity enjoyed in the spirit of recreation and as an integral part of practical daily life, created individuals who were actively in touch with their environment rather than passive observers.

Today, in an effort to match the pace and pressure of modern life, we have abandoned many of the aspects that contribute to a healthy life at home and in the workplace. Frozen dinners, and instant and refined foods have reduced cooking from an art to a mere exercise, robbing individuals, families, and ultimately society of their biological strength. Instead of a traditional diet based on complex carbohydrates, beans, and fresh vegetables, the modern diet is based around animal protein, saturated fats, and refined sugars.

The information age has spawned a new generation of sedentary jobs which many attempt to balance with excessive amounts of vigorous exercise. Without strong cooking to regulate this hectic pace, we move from one extreme to another, never feeling quite healthy enough or free from worry. In striving to make life more convenient, we shrink from pressures and difficulties because we have lost the vitality to overcome them.

The Levels of Stress

The general tendency today is to associate stress-related problems solely with factors outside of ourselves, or "out of our control." It is true that many aspects of modern life are stressful and may contribute to the pressures we experience. Living in overcrowded cities and unventilated buildings, wearing synthetic clothing, being surrounded by machinery and excessive noise add to the burden. Economic factors such as living on credit, taking on a mortgage, or holding an unfulfulling job create demands many fear they will be unable to meet. Perhaps paramount is the fear of nuclear war and the destruction of the natural environment.

The notion that these factors are primarily responsible for stress-related problems is reinforced by the growing separation, or lack of rhythm, between our lifestyles and our sense of unity with nature and the universe. At the root of this alienation is a disorderly way of life, including the habitual practice of improper diet and lack of balance in mental, emotional, and physical activities.

Generally speaking, we can summarize the varieties of stress into the following four categories:

1. *Physical Stress:* A feeling of tension caused by physical hardness in the muscles, joints, blood vessels, and tissues resulting in rigidity and a lack of bodily flexibility.

2. *Emotional Stress:*   Problems in maintaining satisfying and fulfilling relationships with others, as well as a confident self-image, due to our preoccupation with abnormal emotions such as fear, worry, and anxiety.

3. *Intellectual and Social Stress:*   A feeling of helplessness or resignation resulting from the rapid exchange and development of information, and by the sheer magnitude of accumulated data in the modern world.

   Also contributing to this type of stress are the social pressures and frustrations in accepting the pace of change in society at large, especially the separation of families, crime, the threat of nuclear war, and the energy, ecological, and economic crises.

4. *Spiritual Stress:*   Stress caused by the difficulty in coping with the changing universe, including the ability to resolve such basic questions as life and death, sickness and health, and the ephemerality of human existence.

Underlying these forms of stress is a diet and way of life that is separate from the natural order. In the twentieth century the traditional diet of whole grains and fresh, local vegetables has been replaced by meat, cheese, and other animal products, refined sugar, white flour, and mass-produced, artificial foods. The overconsumption of animal food produces a condition of hardness and inflexibility, leading to tension and rigidity in body and mind. With this condition as a base, it is more difficult to adapt to our ever-changing environment, including changes in society.

The breakdown of the family in modern times has also paralleled the shift from traditional patterns of eating and is a major factor in the stressful environment in the modern world. The pre-industrial family was nourished by traditional agricultural products and experienced a sense of unity and cohesion. Today, family members are often isolated from one another, and they lack the network of family members and friends to help them deal with the ups and downs of life.

When our lives are more in harmony with nature we feel connected to its timeless rhythms of day and night, the changing seasons, and the normal cycle of life from birth, to growth, to maturity and old age. It is through this natural contact that we develop faith in the order of the universe and are able to resolve the most basic questions of human destiny. The macrobiotic way of life helps each of us to establish the connection and begin living as a part of the infinite universe and its order.

Stress, Hypertension, Yin and Yang————————————————

In order to understand stress and hypertension, we must see their most basic causes. The principle of yin and yang can be an invaluable tool in helping us to develop this understanding.

Stress and hypertension caused by excessive yang: These disorders are caused by too much inward force or downward pressure. Consequently, this type of stress results when we feel the pressures of daily life closing in around us. To illustrate, we may use the example of a pressure cooker. As the cooker is heated the steam generated will continue to build pressure until it escapes through the release valve. As individuals, it is our flexibility that allows us to balance such pent-up pressures.

Stress from a yang cause becomes unmanageable when the muscles, tissues, and organs become hard and the flow of energy becomes stagnant. Such a condition results when we include a large amount of meat, eggs, or other animal food high in saturated fat in our diet. These types of hard fats rob our bodies of their physical flexibility. If the brain cells and especially the mid-brain also becomes hard, our thinking often becomes rigid and narrow, and we behave more aggressively and egocentrically toward the outer world. Our circulatory system is affected in the same way as the arteries and veins—normally flexible (open) and elastic,—which become clogged and narrow by deposits of fat and cholesterol. The result is often high blood pressure, as the heart struggles to pump blood through increasingly smaller passages.

In general, we become more susceptible to stress and hypertension from a yang cause as our bodies, and eventually our way of thinking, become rigid, narrow, and inflexible due to the overconsumption of more yang foods, especially animal products that are high in saturated fats. However, even within the range of whole, natural foods, this type of stress can result from too many baked flour products, excess salt, or from a lack of freshness and variety in our diets.

Stress and hypertension caused by excessive yin: These disorders result from outward pressure caused by overexpansion. A common example takes place when we inflate a balloon. The surface of the balloon becomes hard and tight as the air pressure inside increases. If we continue to add air, the balloon will burst. This type of stress also causes a lack of flexibility as the outward pressure on tissues, vessels, and organs causes them to become stretched and taut, like an inflated balloon.

Stress from a yin cause increases as we take a larger volume of sugar, fluid, tropical fruits and juices, and raw foods. These types of yin foods cause bodily structures to expand and the volume of blood to increase. As these tendencies become excessive, blood vessels can be stretched to their breaking point. A stroke caused by the eruption of blood vessels in the brain is an extreme example of this condition. Our circulatory system can also become weak when a swollen heart can not adequately pump the increased volume of blood throughout the body. The result is often high blood pressure.[1]

The effect of yin stress on our personalities can be dramatic. As we begin to lose our physical strength and sense of direction, we anger easily over petty problems and frustrations. We may also react violently to any strong stimulus from our surroundings, just as the slightest prick will cause the balloon to burst.

In general, this category of stress or hypertension occurs when we consume more extremely yin foods. Among whole, natural foods, it can also arise if we take too many desserts, too much liquid, raw foods, oil, or spices. Overeating and poor chewing are also important contributing factors. The table below summarizes the primary causes of stress and hypertension from yin and yang causes.

Yin and Yang Causes of Stress and Hypertension

Yin	Yang
Pressure from inside out	Pressure from outside in
Caused by over-expansion	Caused by over-contraction
Primary food causes (when consumed in excess):	Primary food causes (when consumed in excess):
Sugars, liquid, tropical fruit, spices, alcohol, coffee, milk, ice cream, chemicals, drugs, medications.	Meat, eggs, poultry, hard salty cheese, seafood, salt.

Stress Prevention Begins at an Early Age ─────

As adults, we must look not only at our present condition and those factors, dietary and otherwise, that contribute to a stressful way of life. It is equally important to see how the progressive accumulation of these factors from childhood, through adolescence and into maturity have reduced our ability to harmonize our lives and the lives of our children and families with nature, and with life in modern society.

As we have seen, physical hardness and rigidity lead to a lack of flexibility in body and mind. This condition not only causes us to lose touch with nature but also engenders a feeling of separation from family members and friends. Children do not usually experience these feelings. Because their physical conditions are soft and flexible, they easily adapt to changing situations at home, school, and in the social environment of their peers. Thus, flexibility in body and mind is associated with such child-like attributes as a vivid imagination, creativity, open mindedness, playfullness, optimism, and honesty.

Lack of flexibility and feelings of isolation from our physical and social surroundings usually begin after childhood as stagnation and hardness appear in the body. When we eat excessive amounts of cheese, milk, butter, eggs, poultry, meat, and other foods containing heavy saturated fats, together with sugar, ice cream, tropical fruits and drinks, and refined or processed foods, we lose our awareness of the changing natural environment. Deposits of hard fat begin to form in the arteries, blood vessels, and in and around the organs. Tissues become rigid rather than flexible and the skin becomes hard, rough, and insensitive.

Nine out of ten adults have this condition to one degree or another. It can be diagnosed by lying on your back, knees raised and feet flat on the floor. Slowly breath out and press into your lower abdomen deeply, but gently, with the extended fingers of both hands. If you feel hardness or pain, the tissues in this region have already been affected.

As our physical condition becomes more rigid, our thinking, emotions, and outlook reflect this change. Creativity and originality are replaced by imitation and lack of imagination. Instead of being open-minded and full of curiosity, our view becomes narrow and closed, while optimism and honesty may change into negativity and the repression of our thoughts and feelings. All too often love and warmth are replaced by coldness and detachment. Our expression can take the form of criticizing, scolding, or belittling others while frustration builds as we lose the ability to freely express ourselves.

The principles of macrobiotic family life are designed to counteract this destructive trend. The understanding and practice of natural diet, with home cooking as the basis for family health and well-being, combined with a respect for nature and the changing environment can foster a flexible outlook from an early age, and enable us to deal effectively with mature social adaptation.

Within and Without: Balancing Our Internal and External Environments

The quality of our daily life is inseparable from the quality of our environment. Air, water, soil, and sunlight combine to create food that we take in through our digestive system, while other vibrations, radio waves, cosmic rays, and numerous other energies are constantly received and channeled through our nervous system. Thus, the yang aspect of our daily diet, physicalized food, and the yin aspect, vibration, combine the forces of nature to harmonize body and mind, establishing our connection to the world around us.

In modern times, the traditional, balanced diet of whole grains, beans, and fresh vegetables has been replaced with meat, poultry, and other overly yang foods in combination with sugar, spices, and other extreme yin foods. In addition, stressful environmental and social factors have further contributed to an already overburdened system. As a result, our essential and biological connection to nature is often distorted or forgotten.

By beginning to study food selection and preparation using macrobiotic principles, we can regain a sound, natural harmony. As our organs begin to expand and contract in unison, the bodily processes of absorption, assimilation, and elimination proceed unhindered. The constant flow of energy in the form of food and environmental stimuli is taken in, utilized, and released as we become a functioning part of nature as opposed to a mere observer. By adding appropriate physical activity and time for self-reflection, we encourage proper balance between mental, emotional, and physical health. As our condition improves we view what were previously considered stressful situations as challenges to be met creatively, convinced we can attain any goal or accept any outcome as our own responsibility.

As our body adapts to the natural flow of energy we naturally reduce our exposure to electrical devices, fluorescent lights, and high-voltage lines. Cooking on an electric range or in a microwave oven produces undesirable effects that we can now sense, so they are avoided in favor of gas cooking appliances.

Synthetic clothing begins to feel uncomfortable next to our skin and is exchanged for cotton, silk, or linen.

Free circulation of air and direct access to sunlight removes barriers between outside and inside, so our homes and workplaces are adjusted accordingly.

When we eat a more centrally balanced diet, increase our physical activity, and center our thoughts and feelings, we naturally begin to reduce our reliance upon unnecessary technological comforts. While we continue to appreciate and use some of the technological advances modern civilization offers, we seek to reduce our use of excessive electronic or mechanical conveniences that may hinder the smooth exchange of energy between ourselves and our natural environment.

As the distinction between natural and artificial, chaos and harmony, is polarized by our approach to diet and way of life, all our activities express a natural balance of strength and gentleness, endurance and spontaneity, perseverance and flexibility. Harmonizing physical, mental, and emotional, internal and external, unifies us with the order of nature. Life is no longer complicated by stress but made simple by moving to this natural rhythm.

Cooking and Chewing: The Most Profound Forms of Exercise

Exercise can be classified as either physical, mental, or spiritual. The most balanced forms of exercise stimulate all of our physiological systems. Such is the case with cooking and chewing. The thought that goes into menu planning, the physical aspects of preparing and eating, the absence of thought, or empty mind, that occurs when chewing, and the development of spiritual health through the refinement of intuition involved in both cooking and chewing, yield a unique synthesis of all three aspects of the self.

Cutting vegetables, washing grains and beans, carrying spring water, making tofu and seitan, kneading whole-grain bread dough, and similar activities involve the use of a wide range of muscles, joints, and bones. Doing dishes and cleaning up after a meal is a form of physical activity that should be shared regularly by all family members. Any activity that can be performed in a calm, steady way with fluid or circular movements will help unify body and mind.

Chewing utilizes all the muscles of the body and is the key to proper digestion. By contributing to the more efficient utilization of nutrients, chewing is like physical activity in that it increases the proportion of oxygen extracted from the blood. Thus, it is important to chew each mouthful very well, at least fifty times and up to a hundred or more, until the food becomes liquified. When we chew, we should do little else, as peaceful chewing and a peaceful state of mind are synonymous.

When we begin to practice macrobiotic cooking we must think about yin and yang when selecting vegetables and many of us methodically count each chew before swallowing. As our exercise continues we notice that meals come together naturally and only well-chewed food finds its way into our stomachs.

This natural understanding, aided by self-reflection, is unique to macrobiotic education. It is the simple and harmonious approach to our daily food that gradually infuses all aspects of our lives with a sense of balance. In this way all difficulties can be overcome and life can be free of all unnecessary stress.

It has been said that there is only one way to develop our intuition, that is to exercise it. There is no class or book that can provide better instruction in this than that which we provide for ourselves. What could be more simple . . . or more profound?

---

[1] A more detailed explanation of the development of heart disease as well as research conducted by Harvard University showing the effectiveness of the macrobiotic diet in lowering blood pressure and cholesterol levels is presented in *Diet for A Strong Heart*, by Michio Kushi and Alex Jack. St. Martins Press, 1985.

3. Explanation of the Standard Macrobiotic Diet with Dietary Adjustments for Stress and Hypertension ▬▬▬

Below are general dietary recommendations suggested for individuals in a sound state of health. Following each category, there are adjustments for those experiencing stress and/or hypertension from a more yang cause, and one's for those experiencing stress and/or hypertension from a more yin cause. For those experiencing imbalance from both extremes, it is best to eat more centrally, including a wide variety of foods, but avoiding items which are either more expansive (yin), or contractive (yang).

In some cases, further modifications of diet may be appropriate, and for this we recommend seeing a qualified macrobiotic teacher. Also persons with serious illness are advised to consult with the appropriate medical or nutritional professionals in addition to macrobiotic practice.

It should be noted that this is a general guideline, and regardless of your condition, your individuality, life style, and environment need to be taken into account and your diet adapted accordingly.

To see which foods are recommended, refer to the food list following this section.

WHOLE CEREAL GRAINS.   It is recommended that at least 50 percent of every meal include cooked, organically grown, whole cereal grains prepared in a variety of ways. This includes short-grain rice, medium- and long-grain rice, barley, millet, oats, wheat, rye, whole corn, buckwheat, pearl barley, and sweet rice.

Cracked grains may also be eaten from time to time, including bulgur, couscous, steel-cut oats, rolled oats, corn grits, wheat and rye flakes, and cracked wheat.

Flour products such as noodles, pasta, *fu*, and *seitan*, as well as breads, pancakes, muffins, tortillas, crepes, and waffles made from whole grain flours can be enjoyed occasionally. Please note that we do not recommend using either yeasted or baking powder breads, but we do use natural-rise sourdough for leavening in flour products.

Adjustments for stress and/or hypertension from a more yang cause.
Choose primarily whole grains and emphasize short-grain and medium-grain rice. Barley and pearl barley can also be eaten frequently. All

the other whole grains can be enjoyed for variety with the exception of buckwheat. Buckwheat is a more yang grain and should only be eaten on occasion if desired.

Grains can be pressure-cooked or boiled and served in a variety of ways. Grain dishes can be cooked with a small amount of sea salt or *kombu* sea vegetable. On occasion, miso, *tamari* soy sauce, or *umeboshi* plum can be used in cooking. Rice vinegar, *mirin*, parsley, scallions, and celery leaf can also be used for seasoning.

Though you will mostly be using whole grains, you can also include whole grain pasta, wheat noodles (*udon*), cracked grains like bulgur and rolled oats, seitan (wheat gluten) and fu for variety. Noodles made from buckwheat flour are best avoided until your condition becomes more balanced.

Natural-rise sourdough flour products like whole grain breads, pancakes, and muffins, as well as unleavened cookies and pastries can be used occasionally. It is best to limit your intake of these foods as too much flour can inhibit your body's ability to change and heal itself (especially baked flour).

Adjustments for stress and/or hypertension from a more yin cause.
Using primarily whole grains, emphasize short-grain rice, using millet as a secondary grain. Also include all of the other whole grains, using less corn and pearl barley. (These are more yin grains.)

Regularly pressure-cook grains and also include a variety of other cooking styles. Seasoning can include sea salt, umeboshi plum, miso, and tamari soy sauce. These can be used moderately; one pinch of sea salt per cup of grain, for example.

Whole wheat noodles and pasta, buckwheat noodles (*soba*), cracked cereal grains and grain products like bulgar and rolled oats can be used for variety. Seitan, *mochi*, and fu can also be included. Mochi is especially good pan-fried or baked and eaten in miso soup.

Occasionally, whole grain sourdough breads, muffins, and the like, can be eaten, as well as unleavened cookies and pastries. (As long as they are not too sweet.) Again, too much flour, especially baked flour with oil and/or sweetener can really inhibit your progress.

SOUPS.   Approximately 5 to 10 percent of your daily food (one or two bowls daily), may include soup made with traditional and naturally processed miso or tamari soy sauce. The flavor should not be overly salt, and your soups may include a variety of grains, beans, and vegetables, including sea vegetables such as *wakame* and kombu. A small amount of fresh garnish can be eaten with each serving; examples include scallion, parsley, ginger, watercress, and so on.

Other garnishes like *nori* strips, sesame seeds, carrot flowers, and red radish slices can also be used.

Adjustments for stress and/or hypertension from a more yang cause. One bowl of soup can be eaten daily and seasoned with barley miso or tamari soy sauce most often. Umeboshi plum, sea salt, and lighter miso can also be used for variety. The taste of soups can be more light and sweet, rather than salty.

Leafy greens and white vegetables can be used frequently in soups, as can *shiitake* mushrooms. A wide variety of other vegetables, grains, beans, noodles, and sea vegetables (wakame, kombu, and dulse) can also be used.

Most of the time your soups can be lighter and cooked a shorter time, but on occasion a long-time simmered, rich, hearty soup can be eaten.

Each bowl of soup can be garnished with fresh green scallions, parsley, celery leaf, chives, or ginger. Other garnishes like nori.strips, carrot flowers, and toasted sesame seeds can be used in combination with these.

Adjustments for stress and/or hypertension from a more yin cause. One or two bowls of miso or tamari broth soups can be eaten daily. Three-year barley miso (*mugi* miso) can be used most often as a seasoning. Other miso, like soybean miso (*Hatcho*), brown rice miso (*genmai*), and lighter miso (white miso, yellow miso, chick-pea miso, etc.) can be used on occasion for variety. (You can use the darker miso more often.) Umeboshi plum and sea salt can also be used to season a soup.

The taste of soup can be moderate, not too salty, and root, ground, and sea vegetables can be used frequently in making soups. Other vegetables, beans, grains, and noodles can be used to create a wide variety of different soups. Pan-fried (with or without oil) or baked mochi can be eaten frequently in miso soup for increased strength and vitality.

Many different cooking styles can be used in making soup—long-time simmered, short-time cooked, pressure-cooked, sautéed, and so on. Each bowl of soup can be garnished with chopped scallion, parsley, ginger, chive, celery leaf, and nori, carrot, sesame seeds, bonita flakes, and the like.

BEANS AND BEAN PRODUCTS. Approximately 5 percent of your daily diet may include cooked beans and bean products. These include *azuki* beans, chick-peas, lentils, black soybeans, kidney beans, navy beans, lima beans, black beans, split peas, and others, as well as *tofu, tempeh*, dried tofu and *natto*.

Whole beans can be cooked with sea vegetables like kombu to enhance their digestability. They can be pressure-cooked or boiled, and seasoned with sea salt, and miso, tamari soy sauce, umeboshi plum, scallions, parsley, or rice vinegar. Beans can be prepared in a variety of ways—as soup, with grain, in stews, as a side dish with or without other vegetables, in noodle dishes, and so on.

Bean products like tempeh, tofu, dried tofu, *yuba*, *okara*, and natto can be used on occasion and prepared in a number of different ways. Fu and seitan (mentioned in the section on grains), can also be used as bean products in cooking because they contain so much protein.

Adjustments for stress and/or hypertension from a more yang cause. Using primarily azuki beans, chick-peas, lentils, and black soybeans, also include a wide variety of other beans. Beans can be cooked with sea vegetables like wakame or kombu and sea salt. They can be used in a variety of dishes, and can be either boiled or pressure-cooked. Seasoning can include tamari soy sauce, miso, or umeboshi plum, and the taste should be light. Beans can be garnished with chopped scallions, parsley, celery leaf, or chives. Occasionally, the can be flavored with rice vinegar.

Bean products like tempeh, tofu, natto, and okara can be used from time to time and cooked in a variety of ways. Raw tofu can also be used occasionally—in salad dressings, pickled, or marinated, for example.

Fu and seitan can be used occasionally cooked into soups, stews, noodle broth, or vegetable dishes.

Adjustments for stress and/or hypertension from a more yin cause. Use primarily azuki beans, lentils, chick-peas and black soybeans. Beans can be cooked in a wide variety of dishes and can be pressure-cooked, boiled, and sometimes baked. Wakame or kombu and sea salt can be used in cooking. Beans can be seasoned with miso, tamari soy sauce, or umeboshi plum.

Of all the bean products, fresh tofu is the most yin and can be used less often. (Raw tofu can be avoided until your condition changes.) Seitan and fu, along with the other bean products, can be used from time to time for variety. Seitan stew with root vegetables is especially helpful here.

VEGETABLES. Approximately 25 to 30 percent of daily meals are comprised of fresh vegetables. This category includes root vegetables (carrot, burdock, *daikon*, radish, rutabaga, onion, etc.), ground vegetables (cauliflower, broccoli, cabbage, winter squash, leeks, yellow squash, peas, etc.), and leafy greens (carrot tops, kale, mustard greens, watercress, daikon leaves, collard greens, dandelion greens, etc.).

Vegetables can be cooked in a variety of ways including steaming, boiling, par-boiled, light or long-time sauté, nishime style (waterless), baked, broiled, deep-fried, or pickled. They can be used to create an endless variety of dishes like lightly boiled salads, rich root-vegetable stews, *tempura*, salads, and crispy pickles. Vegetables are also frequently cooked in soups, with grains, beans, with sea vegetables, and in desserts.

Sea salt, miso, tamari soy sauce, umeboshi plum, paste, and vinegar, rice vinegar, mirin, ginger, sesame oil, and lemon juice are among some of the seasonings that can be used with vegetables. If you are using seasonings, use them so that they enhance the natural flavor of foods rather than hiding them.

Adjustments for stress and/or hypertension from a more yang cause.
Although a wide range of vegetables, including root, ground, and leafy varieties, can be eaten, emphasis should be placed on sweet, ground vegetables and leafy, green vegetables. Daikon, dried daikon, daikon greens, and shiitake mushrooms are especially helpful.

All styles of cooking can be used, including lighter styles of cooking more often—like boiling, steaming, par-boiling, pressed salad, and quick pickles. Raw salad can also be eaten on occasion if desired. Salty seasonings like sea salt, tamari soy sauce, miso, and umeboshi plum can be kept to a minimum when cooking vegetables. More yin seasonings like mirin and rice vinegar can be used for variety. A small amount of light sesame or dark sesame oil can be used in cooking a few times a week if desired.

Adjustments for stress and/or hypertension from a more yin cause.
Here, also, a wide variety of vegetables can be eaten. Emphasis can be placed more on sweet, ground vegetables and root vegetables. Burdock, lotus root, dried daikon, carrots, cabbages, and winter squash are especially helpful.

All styles of cooking can be used, using the longer styles of cooking often. (Please note that it is also important to have lightly cooked, leafy green vegetables daily.) Nishime style and *kinpira* style of cooking can be used often.

Seasoning can include sea salt, miso, tamari soy sauce, umeboshi plum, and sauerkraut. Rice vinegar, mirin, ginger, scallions, toasted sesame seeds, and so on, can also be used on occasion if desired. Toasted sesame oil can also be used a few times a week in cooking.

Use seasonings to draw out the natural flavor of foods rather than overwhelming them.

SEA VEGETABLES. Approximately 5 percent of daily food can include sea vegetables. These include *hijiki, arame,* kombu, wakame, nori, dulse, agar-agar, kelp, alaria, sea palm, laver (whole nori), Irish moss, and *mekabu.* Sea vegetables can be prepared in a variety of ways: in soups, grain dishes, with beans, in condiments, in desserts, vegetable dishes, salads, and as a side dish by themselves.

Every day, a small amount of sea vegetables can be used in cooking, and a few times a week, a small sea-vegetable side dish, seasoned with tamari soy sauce or other seasoning, can be eaten.

Adjustments for stress and/or hypertension from a more yang cause.
Aside from using sea vegetables daily in cooking, a small sea-vegetable side dish can be made a few times a week. Hijiki, arame, kombu, wakame, nori, and sea palm can all be used. They can be cooked alone or with other vegetables. Tofu, dried tofu, tempeh, and fu can also be cooked with sea vegetables. If desired, a small amount of rice vinegar, mirin, ginger, scallions, or toasted seeds can be added for variety. Sea vegetables can be boiled, or sautéed and boiled, and some sea vegetables can be steamed. Miso or umeboshi plum can also be used as an occasional seasoning instead of tamari soy sauce. Remember, all salty seasoning should be light rather than salty tasting.

Adjustments for stress and/or hypertension from a more yin cause.
A person with a more yin condition can follow basically the same suggestions as above, except seasoning can be a little stronger. Hijiki cooked with root vegetables is especially helpful.

Supplementary Foods ━━━━━━━━━━━━━━━━━━━━━━━━━━

SEEDS AND NUTS. A wide variety of more local, less-fatty seeds and nuts can be used in cooking or as a snack. These include whole sesame seeds, sunflower seeds, pumpkin seeds, squash seeds, almonds, walnuts, filberts, peanuts, and pecans. All seeds and nuts can be toasted before eating, and remember that a little goes a long way.

It is best to refrain from eating seed and nut butters until one's condition becomes more clean and balanced.

Adjustments for stress and/or hypertension from a more yang cause.
Primarily using seeds, such as sesame seeds or pumpkin seeds, the use of seeds and nuts can be minimized. Occasionally, a small amount of toasted seeds or nuts can be used in cooking or eaten as a snack.

Adjustments for stress and/or hypertension from a more yin cause.
Sesame and pumpkin seeds can be used most often, keeping other seeds and nuts to a minimum. All seeds and nuts are oily and if too

much are eaten, they can really slow down your progress. If a small amount is desired for a snack, they can be roasted and seasoned with a little tamari soy sauce or sea salt.

FISH.   A few times a week, a small amount of fresh, white-meat fish can be eaten if desired. This includes sole, halibut, haddock, flounder, cod, fresh-water trout, shrimp, oysters, scallops, and other white-meat fish.

Fish can be cooked in a variety of ways: fish soup or stew, baked fish, stuffed fish, broiled fish, *sushi*, kabobs, salad, and so on. All fish dishes can be served with a condiment to help balance and digest the animal food. Grated daikon with a drop of tamari soy sauce is used most often, but ginger, scallion, lemon, and horseradish can also be used. When fish is served with a meal, plenty of leafy green vegetables can also be included.

Adjustments for stress and/or hypertension from a more yang cause.
As fish is a more yang food, it is best to eat less until your condition becomes more balanced. If desired, a small amount of fish can be eaten on occasion. It is best to prepare fish in a more yin style, like steaming, poaching, or in soup. In a meal where fish is served, make sure there are also plenty of vegetables, especially leafy greens, and a condiment suitable for balancing fish.

Adjustments for stress and/or hypertension from a more yin cause.
A few times a week a small amount of white-meat fish can be eaten. Fish can be cooked in a variety of ways, including broiling, baking, and as tempura. Fish can be seasoned with sea salt, miso, or tamari soy sauce, along with other seasonings. Fish dishes can be served with a small amount of grated daikon and tamari soy sauce condiment, or another condiment suitable for fish—horseradish, ginger, lemon, and the like.

DESSERTS.   A few times a week, a dessert made from whole grains, beans, vegetables and/or fruits can be enjoyed. This includes squash pudding, apple pie, fruit gelatins (*kanten*), *amazaké* pudding, whole grain cookies, fresh fruit, and many more.

For sweeteners, whole grain syrups are used, like rice syrup or barley malt. Fresh fruits, fruit juices, amazake, raisins, and other dried fruits, and sweet vegetables can also be used as sweeteners in desserts. Whole grain flours and cold-pressed oils can be used in baking, *kuzu* and arrowroot as thickeners, agar-agar as gelatin, and seeds and nuts can also be added on occasion.

Adjustments for stress and/or hypertension from a more yang cause.

A few times a week you can make dessert using grains, beans, vegetables and/or fruits. Desserts can be more mild or sweetened with one of the sweeteners mentioned in the previous paragraph. It is better to choose desserts that are lighter (fruit kanten, or gelatin, squash pudding, amazake, etc.), rather than desserts that are heavier (cookies, pastries, etc.).

If you are constantly craving sweets and/or have a tendency toward hypoglycemia, it is best to satisfy your sweet tooth with sweet vegetables rather than other desserts. The azuki, kombu, and squash dish, sweet-vegetable juice, corn on the cob, winter squash, cooked daikon, and cooked onions are some of the dishes with a more sweet taste.

Adjustments for stress and/or hypertension from a more yin cause.
As desserts and sweets are generally more yin, it is better to satisfy your desire for sweets with sweet grains and vegetables. Millet and squash soup, the azuki, kombu, and squash dish, nishime-style vegetables, mochi, and carrot and burdock kinpira are some of the sweeter dishes.

If craved, desserts with whole grains, beans, and/or vegetables with grain sweeteners rather than desserts made with fruit are better. These include squash pudding, amazake kuzu, mochi with rice syrup, and rice pudding.

SEASONINGS. A variety of different seasonings are used in macrobiotic cooking. These include miso, tamari soy sauce, sea salt, umeboshi plums, umeboshi paste, umeboshi vinegar, rice vinegar, sweet rice vinegar, mirin, *saké*, rice syrup, barley malt, scallions, parsley, ginger, and onions.

There are many different brands of miso, tamari soy sauce, and sea salt. It is important to obtain the best quality available. Choose miso that is unpasteurized and organic. When looking for barley miso (mugi miso), for daily use, choose that which has been aged for two to three years. Tamari soy sauce can be made with wheat, soybeans, and sea salt. It should be aged naturally for at least two years. Sea salt can also vary in quality and can be too refined or not refined enough. The color of sea salt should be white, off-white, or very light grey. Make sure you buy cold-pressed, unfiltered oils and check to make sure they are not rancid. Corn and light sesame oil should have a light, sweet smell, and toasted sesame oil can have a slightly sweet, bitter smell. If oil has an acrid smell it is probably rancid and should not be eaten.

BEVERAGES. Any traditional tea which does not have an aromatic fragrance or stimulant effect can be used, such as *bancha* stem tea, roasted grain teas, dandelion root coffee and chickory. You can also drink a moderate amount of spring water. Please refer to the food list in the next section for more beverage ideas.

It is best to drink only when thirsty and to avoid drinking either very cold or very hot beverages.

Adjustments for stress and/or hypertension from a more yang cause. In addition to the above, beverages from the occasional- or infrequent-use columns of the food list can be taken from time to time. Sweet-vegetable juice (see recipe) can be especially helpful.

Adjustments for stress and/or hypertension from a more yin cause. It is best to avoid over-drinking as well as beverages from the infrequent-use list.

SNACKS.   It is best to eat two to three meals each day on a regular schedule. If desired, a small amount of snack food can be eaten also. Some of these foods are: leftovers from another meal, rice balls, rice sushi, noodle sushi, rice cakes, popcorn, mochi, toasted seeds or nuts —alone or with a small amount of dried fruit—noodles and broth (or another noodle dish), sourdough bread, vegetables with a tofu dip, and so on. Bean and/or vegetable dips and spreads can also be easily made to go with vegetables, bread, or rice cakes. Sweet vegetables, like winter squash or corn on the cob also make good snacks.

A More Detailed Macrobiotic Food List ─────────

Grains: ──────────────────────────────────

Regular Use	Occasional Use	Occasional Flour Products
Short-grain brown rice	Long-grain brown rice	Whole wheat noodles
Medium-grain brown rice	Sweet brown rice	Udon noodles
Barley	Mochi	*Somen* noodles
Pearl barley	Cracked wheat, bulgur	Soba noodles (buckwheat)
Millet	Steel-cut oats	Unyeasted whole wheat bread
Whole grain corn	Rolled oats	Unyeasted rye bread
Corn on the cob (in season)	Corn grits	Fu
Whole oats	Cornmeal	Seitan
Whole wheat berries	Rye flakes	
Buckwheat	Couscous	
Rye		

Vegetableg:

Regular Use	Occasional Use	Avoid
Acorn squash	Celery	Artichoke
Bok choy	Chives	Bamboo shoots
Broccoli	Coltsfoot	Beets
Broccoli rabe	Cucumber	Curley dock
Brussels sprouts	Endive	Eggplant
Burdock	Escarole	Fennel
Buttercup squash	Green beans	Ferns
Butternut squash	Green peas	Ginseng
Cabbage	Iceberg lettuce	Green and red peppers
Carrots and their tops	Jerusalem artichoke	New Zealand spinach
Cauliflower	Kohlrabi	Okra
Chinese cabbage	Lambsquarters	Plantain
Collard greens	Mushrooms	Purslane and shepard's
Daikon and greens	Patty pan squash	purse
Dandelion root and	Romaine lettuce	Potato
greens	Salsify	Sorrel
Hubbard squash	Shiitake mushrooms	Spinach
Hokkaido pumpkin	Snap beans	Sweet potato
Jinenjo	Snow peas	Swiss chard
Kale	Sprouts	Tomato
Leeks	Summer squash	Taro potato (albi)
Lotus root	Wax beans	Yams
Mustard greens		Zucchini
Onions		
Parsley		
Parsnip		
Pumpkin		
Radish		
Red cabbage		
Rutabaga		
Scallions		
Turnip and greens		
Watercress		

Beans:

Regular Use	Occasional Use	Occasional Bean Substitutes
Azuki beans	Black-eyed peas	Dried tofu
Black soybeans	Black turtle beans	Fresh tofu
Chick-peas (garbanzos)	Great northern beans	Natto
Lentils (green)	Jacobs cattle beans	Okara
	Kidney beans	Tempeh

Lima beans   Yuba
Mung beans
Navy beans
Pinto beans
Red lentils
Soybeans
Split peas
Whole dried peas

Sea Vegetables:

Regular Use
Arame
Hijiki
Kombu
Nekombu
Nori
Nori flakes
Dulse
Wakame
Sea palm
Agar-agar
Irish moss
Mekabu

Other Sea Vegetables
(These may be used in addition to regular-use sea vegetables and cannot always be substituted for regular-use sea vegetables in medicinal cooking)
Alaria
Kelp
Fu-nori
Wild nori (laver)

Fruits (usually cooked or dried):

Occasional Use
Apples
Apricots
Blueberries
Blackberries
Cantaloupes
Cherries
Currents
Grapes
Lemons (small amounts of juice for cooking)
Nectarines
Peaches
Pears
Plums
Raisins
Raspberries
Strawberries
Tangerines (small amounts of juice for cooking)

Avoid
Avocados
Bananas
Coconuts
Dates
Figs
Grapefruit
Kiwi fruit
Oranges
Mangoes
Papayas
Persimmons
Pineapple
All other tropical fruits

Honeydew melon
Watermelon

Seeds and Nuts: ————————————————————————————

Occasional Use	*Avoid*
Almonds	Brazil nuts
Chestnuts	Caraway seeds
Filberts	Cashews
Peanuts	Hazelnuts
Pumpkin seeds	Macadamia nuts
Sesame seeds	Pistachios
Sunflower seeds	Poppy seeds
Walnuts	Spanish peanuts
Squash seeds	All tropical nuts
Black sesame seeds	
Alfalfa seeds (as sprouts)	

Animal Foods: ————————————————————————————

Occasional Use	*Avoid*
Carp	Red-meat fish
Clams	Chicken
Cod	All fowl
Crab	All eggs
Flounder	All dairy products
Haddock	
Halibut	
Iriko	
Lobster	
Oysters	
Octopus	
Shrimp	
Scrod	
Sole	
Squid	
Sea bass	
Freshwater trout	
Other white-meat fish	

Pickles: ————————————————————————————

Regular Use	*Avoid*
Bran pickles	Commercial dill pickles
Brine pickles	Herb pickles
Miso bran pickles	Garlic pickles
Miso pickles	Spiced pickles
Pressed pickles	Apple-cider vinegar pickles

Sauerkraut
Tamari pickles
Takuan pickles
Umeboshi pickles

Wine vinegar pickles
All pickles with sugar or
   chemicals

Sweets:

Regular Use	*Occasional Use*	*Avoid*
Cabbage	Amazaké	All tropical fruits
Carrots	Barley malt	Brown sugar
Corn on the cob	Chestnuts	Carob
(in season)	Fruits (see fruit list)	Chocolate
Daikon	Hot apple cider	Fructose
Onions	Hot apple juice	Honey
Parsnips	Rice malt syrup	Maple syrup
Pumpkin		Molasses
Squash		Sorgum
		White sugar

Beverages:

Regular Use	*Occasional Use*	*Infrequent Use*	*Avoid*
Bancha twig tea	Grain coffee	Green tea	Distilled water
(*Kukicha*)	(100% grain)	Vegetable	Coffee
Bancha stem tea	Dandelion tea	juices	Cold, iced drinks
Roasted barley	Kombu tea	Juices of fruits	Carbonated
tea	Umeboshi tea	from fruit list	fruit drinks
Roasted brown	*Mu* tea	Beer	Hard liquor
rice tea	Juice from	Saké	Herb teas
Spring water	cooking		Mineral water
Well water	vegetables		All carbonated
	Amazaké		water
	Roasted corn tea		Regular tea
	Sweet-vegetable		Stimulants
	juice (see recipe)		Sugared drinks
			Tap water
			Whisky
			Wine

Seasonings and Oils:

Regular Use	*Occasional Use*	*Avoid*
Natural miso	Corn oil	Animal fats
Dark sesame oil	Ginger	Butter and cream
Light sesame oil	Horseradish	Coconut oil
Natural soy sauce	Mirin	Cottonseed oil
Tamari soy sauce	Olive oil	Commercial dressings
Unrefined white or	Rice vinegar	Garlic

light gray sea salt
Umeboshi plums and paste
Umeboshi vinegar
Onion
Scallion
Parsley
Celery leaves
Chives

Sweet rice vinegar
Safflower oil
Sunflower oil
Saké lees
Lemon juice
Tangerine juice
Saké
Horseradish
Natural mustard

Linseed oil
Margarine
Mayonnaise
Soybean margarine
Commercial miso
Commercial mustard
Pepper
Peanut oil
Table salt
All commercial seasonings
Soybean oil
Commercial soy sauce
All spices

Condiments:

Main Condiments
Gomashio (sesame salt)
Sea vegetable powders
Sea vegetable powder with roasted sesame seeds
Tekka
Umeboshi plum
Nori flakes
Pickled vegetables
Sauerkraut

Other Condiments
Brown rice vinegar
Cooked miso with scallions and onions
Nori condiment
Roasted shiso leaves
Shiso leaves and roasted sesame seeds
Umeboshi plum with raw scallion or onions
Umeboshi vinegar
Grated daikon with a drop of tamari
Ginger
Shio kombu
Roasted soybeans and miso
Sigure miso relish
Other macrobiotic condiments

Snacks:

The best things to snack on are:
Leftovers
Noodles
Popcorn (unbuttered)
Puffed whole cereal grain
Rice balls
Rice sushi
Noodle sushi
Arepas

Whole wheat sourdough bread
Rice *kayu* bread
Whole wheat rye bread (sourdough)
Homemade bean spreads (hummus, pinto bean spread, tofu dip, etc.)
Carrot spread
Squash spread (Azuki-squash spread)
Onion butter
Apple butter
Rice cakes
Corn on the cob (in season)
Cooked sweet vegetables
Cooked broccoli, cauliflower, etc.
Mochi

Additional Suggestions

You may eat regularly two to three meals per day, as much as you want, provided the proportions are correct and chewing is thorough—at least 50 and as much as 200 times per mouthful, the more the better.

Meals can be eaten in an orderly way. Starting with soup, eat the more yang, heavier dishes first. Then go to the lighter, more yin dishes like leafy greens and salad. Grains can be eaten throughout the meal. Avoid drinking during your meal, as excess liquid can dilute

sleeping.

This may sound like a lot to do, but once put into effect, these suggestions are actually very easy to follow and will make you feel a lot better.

Cooking and Preparation Methods:

Regular Use	Occasional Use
Pressure-cooking	Sautéing
Boiling	Stir-frying
Steaming	Raw
Waterless	Deep-frying
Soup	Tempura
Pickling	Baking
Oilless sautéing (with water)	Broiling
Pressing	
Roasting	

Cooking Aspects to Change for Variety: ————————————
1. Selection of foods within the categories of grains, vegetables, beans, sea vegetables, and so on
2. Methods of cooking
3. Way of cutting vegetables
4. Amount of water used
5. Amount and kind of seasoning and condiments used
6. Tastes of dishes—sweet, bitter, pungent, sour, and so on.
7. Length of cooking time
8. Use of a higher or lower flame
9. Varying the combination of foods and dishes
10. Seasonal cooking adjustments
11. Style of presentation

Way of Life Suggestions and Reminders————————

- Maintain the dream and image of health, peace, and abundance for yourself, others, and the world.
- Live each day happily without being preoccupied with your health, and stay mentally and physically alert and active.
- View everything and everyone you meet with gratitude. Offer thanks before and after each meal.
- It is best to avoid wearing synthetic or woolen clothing directly against the skin. Wear cotton as much as possible, especially for undergarments. Avoid excessive metallic accessories on the fingers, wrists, or neck. Keep such ornaments simple and graceful.
- If your strength permits, go outdoors in simple clothing. Walk on the grass, beach, or soil up to one-half hour every day. Go barefoot when possible.
- Keep your home (and other surroundings) in good order, from the kitchen, bathroom, bedroom, living room, to every corner of the house.
- Initiate and maintain an active correspondence, extending good relationships with everyone around you.
- Avoid taking long hot baths or showers unless you have been consuming too much animal food or salt.
- Scrub your entire body with a hot, damp towel until the skin becomes red, every morning or every night before retiring. If that is not possible, at least scrub your hands, feet, fingers, and toes.
- Avoid chemically perfumed cosmetics. For care of the teeth, brush with natural preparations or sea salt.
- If your condition permits, exercise regularly as part of your daily life, including activities like scrubbing floors, cleaning windows,

and so on, as well as exercise programs such as martial arts, yoga, dance, swimming, soccer, basketball, and so on.

- Avoid using electric cooking devices (ovens or ranges) or microwave ovens. Convert to a gas or wood stove at the earliest opportunity.
- It is best to minimize the use of color television and computer display units.
- Include some large green plants in your house to freshen and enrich the oxygen content of the air in your home.

4. Menu Planning ▬▬▬▬▬▬▬

When planning a menu, there are several things to consider.

1. The relative proportion of grains, vegetables, soup, beans, and so on in a meal as recommended in the Standard Macrobiotic Diet.

2. Make appropriate adjustments for your condition, modifying the standard diet to balance a condition of stress and/or hypertension from either a more yin or more yang cause.

3. Variety in meals. For instance, last night's dinner rice can be this morning's soft rice. It is most important, however, to have fresh soup and fresh, quickly boiled or blanched leafy greens every day. Therefore, boil only as many greens as are needed for one meal. To ensure variety, be sure to consider:

   A. *The types of vegetables and grains used.* Every day have some kind of root vegetable, fresh and leafy greens and, in some form, a small amount of sea vegetable. It is helpful to have brown rice every day, but there are many ways to vary this basic dish as you will see in the menu examples.

   B. *The seasonings, condiments, and pickles used.* (It is preferred that one has a small amount of pickles daily.)

   C. *The cooking methods employed.* Every day, have some quickly boiled or blanched greens, as well as pressure-cooked or longer-time cooked items.

   D. *The sizes, shapes, colors, and textures from dish to dish.* Use attractive garnishes to brighten your meals.

4. *Seasonal and climatic adjustments.* For hot weather, emphasize more fresh, lightly boiled or steamed vegetables, salads, less cooking time, and less oil and salt. For colder weather, emphasize more hearty, rich dishes, stews and thick soups, protein such as found in beans, root vegetables, and a little more salt and oil.

5. *Adjustments for the time of day.* Beans, hardy dishes, and stronger seasonings are best eaten for dinner. It is recommended that lunches and breakfasts be kept simple and light, otherwise one may feel heavy and sluggish throughout the day. Soft porridges and whole-grain cereals are delicious for breakfast.

6. *Adjustments for age.* For babies, younger children, and elderly

persons, serve more soft foods and sweet-tasting vegetables with a minimum amount of seasonings. It is preferred that babies do not eat any salt at all. Teens and adults can have more seasonings and more crisp, solid vegetables.

7. *Life-style adjustments.* People doing more physical exercise, work, and activities need more protein and hardy, rich dishes than do those who are more sedentary.

8. *Use as much of your leftovers as possible.* The menus below disregard leftovers to emphasize variety. Normally, a grain or bean dish, for example, can last for several days or more. Besides simply reheating leftovers, you can rework them into a new format; for instance, last night's dinner rice can be this morning's soft rice. Or you might want to add a few pieces of tofu when heating up yesterday's root vegetables. The possibilities are endless. All this adds more appeal and variety to your meals. It is most important, however, to have fresh, quickly boiled or blanched leafy greens every day. Therefore, boil only as many greens as you can have in one meal.

9. Plan a meal that is reasonable for you to accomplish. At the same time, challenge yourself every day by trying new techniques and dishes. By either trying to make too much, or making only dishes you know well, your cooking experience can be frustrating or boring respectively.

10. When serving meals, vary your presentation by using different serving dishes and a variety of garnishes. Make your food beautiful and your dining area pleasant and clean. Do this even (especially) if you are dining alone.

11. If you eat alone often, consider inviting a friend over to share your meal.

Seven-day Menu Guide

Below is a sample seven-day menu. It is provided as a guide and should be adapted as necessary to meet individual needs. For instance, in order to present as many dishes and ideas as possible, the use of leftovers in the menus has almost been omitted. Remember, however, that you can enjoy the fresh-cooked, energizing kinds of food that you need and still use leftovers in your menu planning. (This can also cut down on cooking time.) For example, one evening for dinner you might make pressure-cooked brown rice, nishime vegetables, and steamed greens among other dishes. Cook extra rice, nishime, and greens. The next morning have soft rice from leftover rice. That afternoon for lunch have rice balls or noodles and broth with leftover nishimi and greens. That evening cook fresh food again, *making sure you are including plenty of variety.*

If this looks a little overwhelming to you, think about this: Day to day, practicing the macrobiotic way of life, you may need to spend more time cooking, exercising, or otherwise taking care of yourself. In the long run, this can be viewed as an investment in abundant health, happiness, and energy. At the same time you can avoid costly medical bills and related troubles from health problems. Macrobiotics is a sane, practical, and economical way of life!

For more ideas and menus, consult the *Complete Guide to Macrobiotic Cooking*, by Aveline Kushi, *The Changing Seasons Macrobiotic Cookbook*, by Aveline Kushi and Wendy Esko, *Macrobiotic Cooking for Everyone*, by Wendy Esko, and *Aveline Kushis' Introducing Macrobiotic Cooking*, by Wendy Esko.

A Seven-day Menu Guide ────────────────────────────────

	BREAKFAST	LUNCH	DINNER
For stress and/or hypertension from a yin cause	Whole oats Toasted whole-wheat bread with onion butter Brine pickles Grain coffee	Soba noodles with vegetable broth Fried tofu Steamed broccoli	Daikon miso soup Pressure-cooked brown rice Azuki, squash, and kombu Boiled salad with kale, celery and carrot flowers with scallion, umeboshi dressing Bancha tea
For stress and/or hypertension from a yang cause	Whole oats Steamed whole-wheat sourdough bread Apple butter Quick pickles Grain coffee	Udon noodles with vegetable broth Fried tofu Steamed broccoli	Daikon-shiitake miso soup Pressure-cooked brown rice Azuki, squash, and kombu Boiled salad with kale, celery and carrot flowers with scallion, umeboshi dressing Bancha tea
For stress and/or	Millet and squash cereal	Noodle sushi Vegetables	Clear broth soup with cauliflower

	BREAKFAST	LUNCH	DINNER
hypertension from a yin cause	*Goma* wakame Barley tea	Pickles	Azuki beans, rice, and sweet rice Scallion-miso condiment Nishime with carrot, rutabaga, onion, kombu and sesame seeds Boiled kale Grain coffee
For stress and/or hypertension from a yang cause	Millet and squash cereal Goma wakame Leftover vegetables Barley tea	Noodle sushi Vegetables Quick pickles	Clear broth soup with cauliflower Azuki beans, rice, and sweet rice Scallion-miso condiment Nishime with carrot, onion, kombu, yellow summer squash, and broccoli Boiled turnip greens Grain coffee Stewed peaches with kuzu
For stress and/or hypertension from a yin cause	Oatmeal with toasted sunflower seeds Bancha tea	Boiled millet and vegetables Steamed bok choy Shio kombu Grain coffee	Fried rice Black soybeans Corn on the cob Kale, cauliflower, and carrots Sauerkraut Stewed dried fruit with kuzu
For stress and/or hypertension from a yang cause	Oatmeal with raisins and toasted sunflower seeds Grain coffee	Boiled barley and vegetables Steamed broccoli rabe Goma wakame Bancha tea	Fried rice Black soybeans Corn on the cob Kale, cauliflower, and carrots Sauerkraut Strawberry kanten
For stress and/or hypertension from a yin cause	Soft-cooked barley with kombu Shiso-leaf condiment Bancha tea	Tempeh sandwich Leftover vegetables Pickles	Miso soup with lotus root, onions, and wakame Rice with corn off the cob Baked trout Daikon and tamari condiment

	BREAKFAST	LUNCH	DINNER
			Boiled kale
			Pressed salad with
			Chinese cabbage,
			red onion, dulse
			radish, and parsley
			Gomashio
			Bancha tea
			Amazaké pudding
For stress and/or hypertension from a yang cause	Soft-cooked barley with kombu Shiso-leaf condiment Bancha tea	Tempeh sandwich Fresh salad Pickles	Corn chowder with fish Boiled medium-grain rice Dried daikon and kombu Boiled kale Pressed salad with Chinese cabbage, red onion, dulse, radish, and parsley Gomashio Bancha tea Amazaké pudding
For stress and/or hypertension from a yin cause	Miso soup Soft rice with umeboshi, nori, and scallions Nuka pickles	Arepas Tempeh and vegetables Boiled watercress Grain coffee	Lentil soup Barley rice Burdock kinpira Baked yellow squash Pressed salad with cabbage, carrot and scallion Nori condiment Bancha tea
For stress and/or hypertension from a yang cause	Miso soup with greens Soft rice with umeboshi, nori, and scallions	Arepas Tempeh and vegetables Boiled watercress Quick pickles Grain coffee	Lentil soup Pearl barley rice Carrot and burdock kinpira Baked yellow squash Pressed salad with lettuce, onion, cucumber, radish, and chickory Nori condiment Bancha tea
For stress and/or hypertension from a yin cause	Soft rice with miso and vegetables Toasted pumpkin seeds	Rice balls Seitan with root vegetables Boiled collard greens	Squash Soup Millet croquettes with kuzu sauce Sautéed hijiki with dried tofu and onions

	BREAKFAST	LUNCH	DINNER
	Dandelion coffee		Boiled salad with broccoli, carrot, and mung-bean sprouts Red radish pickles Bancha tea
For stress and/or hypertension from a yang cause	Soft rice with miso and vegetables Toasted pumpkin seeds Corn tea	Rice salad with seitan Boiled collard greens	Squash soup Millet croquettes with kuzu sauce Sautéed hijiki with fresh tofu and onions Boiled salad with broccoli, carrot, and mung-bean sprouts with rice vinegar Red-radish pickles Bancha tea

	BRUNCH	DINNER
For stress and/or hypertension from a yin cause	Miso soup Buckwheat cream and toast with onion butter or Sourdough pancakes with barley-malt kuzu sauce Scrambled tofu Boiled greens Pickles Grain coffee	Chick-pea rice Arame with carrots and lotus root Chinese-style vegetables Mustard-green pickles Bancha tea
For stress and/or hypertension from a yang cause	Miso soup Soft millet with corn and onions Steamed bread with unsweetened fruit jam or Sourdough pancakes with barley-malt kuzu sauce Scrambled tofu Boiled greens Quick pickles Grain coffee	Chick-pea rice with scallions Arame with carrots and lotus root Chinese-style vegetables Mustard-green pickles Bancha tea

5. Cookware ▬▬▬▬▬▬▬▬▬▬▬▬▬▬▬▬▬▬▬▬▬▬▬

Along with stocking good food, a kitchen needs to be equipped with a collection of essential cookware. Having the right tools at hand frees the mind to work with a more relaxed and creative attitude. This naturally has a profound effect on personal well-being as well as affecting the quality, taste, and appeal of meals. Also, some types of kitchen equipment should best be avoided as they may be detrimental to health, while others are a must for their beneficial influences. Listed below is a checklist of recommended kitchen equipment.

1. We recommend a gas stove as opposed to an electric one. There are several reasons for this:

   A. Electricity dissipates the molecular structure and strength of food by causing the electrons to bounce out of the atomic field, leaving the atom very unstable. Gas, on the other hand, just bounces the molecules around, while leaving them intact.

   B. It is very hard to fine-tune cooking with electricity. It is a conductive heat which first warms the coils and then the pot and its contents from the bottom up. The temperature cannot be changed quickly when turning to high or low because it takes some time to cool or heat the pot. Electricity makes it difficult to cook uniformly and it is possible that ingredients at the bottom of the pan can burn while those at the top need more cooking. A gas flame heats the surrounding air. Food thus cooks much more evenly, and the temperature can be adjusted immediately (a pot of water will instantly stop boiling the moment the flame is turned off, for example). Meals are more well cooked.

   C. Because of these drawbacks in electric cooking, a person may not feel satisfied with the meal and may crave strong salt or animal food (to counter the yin and weakening effects) which in turn causes a craving for excessive sweets and other yin foods. In other words, it becomes more of a struggle to eat in a balanced manner and thus to stay on the macrobiotic diet.

   A microwave oven should be avoided, particularly if a family member is sick. These ovens zap food with radioactive waves at three-billion-cycles per second (an electric stove runs at 60-cycles per second and actually generates a low form of radiation). It disintegrates instead of cooks food, and can cause the same effect in our body. Microwave cooking cannot help in regaining health, and it is suspected to contribute to certain types of illnesses.

After gas, wood is the best source of heat (followed by coal or charcoal) though it is impractical for most modern homes. It has a peaceful energy and at the same time it gives great strength to our foods.

2. Several stainless-steel pots of varying sizes. The steel does not interfere with the energies of the food. It is best to avoid aluminum because it is a poisonous substance and under high temperatures or when cooking very acidic (sweet) or alkaline (salty) foods, harmful toxins are released and mixed in with your ingredients.

   Cookware made out of glass (like Pyrex), earthenware, and enamelware are also excellent materials to cook in. (Be careful that you do not pour cold water into a heated enamel pot or leave it empty over a flame as this will cause it to crack. Let it cool off before washing it. It is also easily scratched so do not clean it with a steel-wool scrubber and use a wooden spoon when handling food inside it.)

3. At least one pressure cooker (stainless or enamel steel). This is an ideal pot for cooking grains, beans, root vegetables (like big chunks of burdock), squash, or anything that takes a long time to soften. The nutrients are better retained and everything is cooked more thoroughly, quickly, and with more energy than when prepared in a regular pot.

Fig. 2   Pressure Cooker

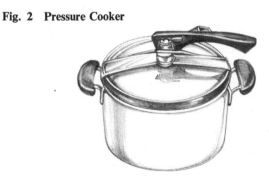

To use, put ingredients inside (not more than ¾ full), cover (don't forget to put the weight attachment on top), and over a medium-high flame, bring to pressure. You can tell the pressure is up when there is a lot of hissing and the weight begins to jiggle and shake. Then, immediately turn down the flame and, if needed, place a heat deflector underneath. Simmer (anywhere from ·5 to 10 minutes to an hour or more depending on what is inside) until the food is done. Take the pot off the stove and let the pressure come down. You can let it come down naturally or rinse the pot under cold running water in the sink. This brings it down right away.

Before you cook, carefully take a good look at the cover. Inspect the hole (on which you place the weight) and make sure that it is not clogged. Otherwise, an explosion can occur when the pressure is high. Also, look at the rubber rings on the inside of the lid and in the pot itself where the rings touch. Remove any bits of food or other substances which may be stuck there as they will create a gap where steam can escape and as a result, the pressure will never build up.

4. Several cast-iron skillets for roasting and sautéing. Season them before their first use and from time to time thereafter. To do this, wash and dry them thoroughly. Then rub sesame oil all over (outside also) with a paper towel. The inside can be coated by rotating and tilting the pan over a flame. Place oiled pans in the oven at 225° to 250° F. for two to three hours. Then, let them sit for a few hours until they cool. Seasoning prevents the pans from rusting. For the same reason, do not soak cast-iron pans in hot, soapy water, and dry them thoroughly over a low flame after washing them.

5. One deep cast-iron pot for deep-frying. Cast iron is the best material to hold the intense heat of the oil.

6. Baking containers including pie plates, bread pans, muffin tins and so on. Again, avoid aluminum.

7. An optional *wok* (a Chinese-style skillet). The cast-iron skillets can effectively cover sautéing needs but a wok is great for light, and fast-cooking vegetables and fish.

8. Several stainless-steel mixing bowls in different sizes for washing and mixing food.

9. Large wooden serving bowls for grains. Wood allows the cooked grains to breathe. It also retards spoilage by absorbing any

excess water. The bowls need to be oiled periodically to prevent them from cracking. Heat some sesame oil, pour it into a completely dry bowl which is rotated until the inside is thoroughly oiled. Oil the outside also, with a brush or paper towel. Let it sit for a few hours until it dries completely.

10. Various other attractive serving containers made of glass, china, or ceramics. (Plastic is to be avoided.)

11. A stainless-steel or bamboo steamer.

12. A colander for rinsing noodles and other foods.

13. A fine-mesh strainer for washing seeds and grains.

14. A *suribachi* and pestle for making gomashio and other condiments. This is a Japanese ceramic bowl with grooves, made for crushing roasted sesame seeds, sea vegetables and so on.

Fig. 3   Suribachi and Pestle

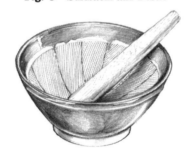

15. A food mill for pureeing cooked grains and vegetables. (An electric blender is more disruptive to the energies of foods. Instead of using one on a regular basis, save it for parties or special occasions when working with large volumes.)

16. A grain mill for grinding grains and nuts into flour. Flour is best when used soon after grinding. After being cracked, grain immediately starts to oxidize, and begins to lose some of its nutrients. Also, it is most delicious when fresh. (A local natural food store may have a good supply of flour as well.)

17. A pickle press for making pickles and pressed salads.

18. An earthenware crock with a wide mouth is good for making bran pickles, among other things.

19. Tea pot or kettle. Avoid aluminum.

20. A tea strainer for straining out leaves and twigs when serving the tea. A bamboo strainer, found in natural food and Oriental stores, is the best one to use.

21. Large glass jars for storing grains, beans, nuts, seeds, and other foods, as well as for making pickles.

22. Wooden cutting boards. Keep a separate one for fish and animal foods as their bacteria can have a toxic effect on vegetables.

23. Knives. The square-shaped Oriental knives are the easiest and the most efficient. They come in:
    A. carbon (which has a good sharp edge but rusts and chips easily),
    B. stainless steel (which does not rust but is not as sharp), and
    C. high-grade carbon with stainless steel which does not rust and is sharp as well (but is more expensive).

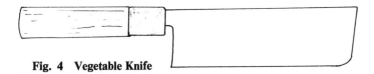

Fig. 4 Vegetable Knife

To protect the carbon knives, as soon as they are used, wash them in warm, soapy water, and then dry them immediately. If rust starts to appear, scrape it off with a steel-wool scrubber. Along with keeping knives as dry as possible, coating them with a little sesame oil after use will provide additional protection.

A sharpening stone will be needed to keep the edges of knifes sharp. Oil the stone with a vegetable oil or rinse it in water before use. Tilt the knife at a twenty-degree angle and sweep the blade against the stone in several circular motions. Use one hand to press down on the blade while the other hand holds the knife and moves it in circles. Sharpen the entire length of the edge. For more control, sharpen just one side (the right side for right handers and the left side for lefties). Do not use this knife for bread as its blade may be destroyed.

24. A bread knife. The best knife for cutting bread has a long, thin blade with a serrated edge.

25. A grater, most often used in macrobiotic cooking for grating fresh ginger, daikon, carrots, onions, lotus root, jinenjo, and taro potato.

26. A vegetable peeler, good for removing skins of cucumbers, apples and so on, when necessary.

27. A flame or heat deflector. This thin metal plate is placed underneath the pot or pressure cooker to even the flame and to help prevent the food from burning. Do not use the white asbestos deflectors as asbestos is poisonous.

28. An oil skimmer for lifting small bits of batter and food from tempura oil as well as for lifting vegetables from a pot of water.

29. A natural-bristle brush for brushing oil into skillets, cookie sheets, muffin tins, pie plates, and so on. Any small, clean, unused brush can be used.

30. Drop tops. These tops fit inside the pot and sit right on top of the food being cooked. This is an especially effective way to cook beans. Drop tops add some pressure but let steam escape and thus the food is cooked more thoroughly and softens more quickly.

31. Drop tops for pickles made in a keg such as bran pickles. A wooden one is best. A heavy stone or weight is placed on top for pressure. A plate is a good substitute if a wooden top cannot be found.

32. Vegetable brushes with natural bristles are best for washing vegetables. They can be found in natural or Oriental food stores.

33. Wooden spoons for stirring, mixing, scooping, and serving food before and after cooking. Wood has the best energy in interaction with food and is gentler to pots, pans, and bowls. Wooden spoons do not scratch cookware.

34. A bamboo rice paddle for handling and serving your grains.

Fig. 5 Rice Paddle

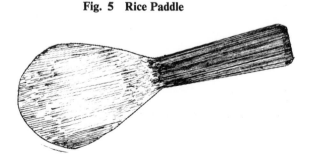

35. Soup ladles.

36. Rubber spatula for scraping batter, puréed food and so on from clean bowls.

37. A metal spatula for turning food over.

38. Cooking chopsticks. These are longer than the table version.

39. A rolling pin.

40. Measuring cups and spoons.

41. Sushi mats for making sushi and for covering cooked food. (They let air circulate and help retard spoilage.)

42. Bamboo mats. Also for covering food.

43. One hundred percent cotton cheesecloths, used as a cover when making pickles and also for making little sacks to contain foods in cooking (sort of like a tea bag).

44. Paper towels.

6. Cooking Attitude

Besides having good-quality food and proper cookware, to be a good cook, the right attitude and frame of mind are also necessary. Here is another check list.

1. A cook should leave all worries, problems, and angers behind as he or she relaxes mind and body into a peaceful, calm state of being. A cook's thoughts and emotions are mixed into the food and have an effect on anyone who eats it. Here are some things, among others, to remember while cooking.

    A. Pour love and healing vibrations into the food, and imagine that whoever eats it will become healthier and happier.

    B. Imagine that the food has the power to help individuals realize their dreams, and that with this tool comes the ability to vitalize and inspire whole civilizations. This is actually true.

    C. Give thanks to the farmer, trucker, storekeeper, nature, the food itself, cookware companies, and anyone else who has made it possible to have these wonderful ingredients and utensils.

    D. A cook can imagine that he or she is composing a symphony or painting a masterpiece as colors, textures, tastes, and smells are arranged into beautiful and dynamic combinations. Anyone who cooks should work to release his or her creativity and intuition. These develop with experience, so be patient and persistent.

    E. Realize that there is always more to learn. One should never become arrogant and think that he or she now knows it all. Be open and learn from everyone. We all have different perspectives and ideas and therefore we all have something to offer.

2. Clean and organize the kitchen and surroundings before, during, and after cooking.

3. Long hair should be tied back to prevent it from catching on fire as well as from falling into the food. Wear a clean apron and roll up long sleeves.

4. Work quickly, calmly, and efficiently, economically making the most of one's time. Avoid munching while cooking as this will really slow things down.

5. Keep other activities and distractions to a minimum and concentrate all energies on the task at hand.

6. When making a menu, first look at all leftovers and older vegetables and use these first. Do not waste any food. Avoid buying more perishables than needed. Check supplies first before going shopping.

7. Develop intuition and common sense in order to appropriately adapt meals to the weather, the season, the people for whom one is cooking, and one's own needs. A cook should be aware of the daily needs and changes of others, his or her own moods, and any other influencing factors for that particular place and time.

8. Keep meals simple. Do not mash together a lot of different ingredients into one dish. Go light on seasonings and use them mainly to draw out and enhance the natural flavors of food.

9. Decorate food beautifully, set the table using appealing tableware, and make the dining area comfortable and aesthetically pleasing. This enhances appetite and the dining experience.

10. Take the time and place to relax, sit down, and peacefully enjoy meals with appreciation. Chew food thoroughly, the saliva helps digestion. Also, it is best not to eat unless one is truly hungry.

7. Grains and Grain Products ▬▬▬

Grains:

Grains stored in a cool, dark, dry location, can be kept indefinitely. Use organically grown grains whenever they are available. To retain their maximum energy, leave grains unhusked until just before cooking, if possible.

Before washing grains, spread a handful at a time on a plate, and remove any stones and other debris which may be mixed in. Then, place the grains in a bowl (lightweight stainless-steel mixing bowls are excellent for this), cover with cold water, and very gently stir and rinse off any dirt that floats to the top. Pour out this water, and repeat the above steps until the water remains clear. Then, place the grain in a colander or strainer. Wash quickly to help retain the grain's nutrients.

There are a variety of grains available:

Brown Rice:

Brown rice, being the easiest to digest, is the most suitable grain for daily use. It can be eaten every day, regardless of whether an individual is in the transitional, healing, or standard phase. We eat brown rice at almost every meal. The other grains serve as variations, either as a substitute or as an additional ingredient in a meal. We mainly use four types of rice:

1. *Short-grain:* Short-grain rice is the variety with the hardiest taste and energy, and the most effective one for creating a healthy, balanced condition. Use this one most of the time, especially in the winter.

2. *Medium-grain:* Medium-grain rice is more soft and moist, and is a nice variation.

3. *Long-grain:* Long-grain rice is light and fluffy, excellent for fried rice, and makes a great alternative in the summer and warmer climates.

4. *Sweet rice:* Sweet rice is even more sweet and glutinous than the short grain, and is quite sticky. Sweet rice can be added to other grains periodically for a sweeter taste, and also serves as a base for *ohagi*, mochi, and amazaké.

We recommend pressure-cooking your rice most of the time. This form of preparation cooks the grains more thoroughly, making them easier to digest. Pressure-cooked grains are less soggy, and are sweeter and more healing. Along with the help of a pressure cooker there are two ways to make your grain softer, sweeter, and more digestible:

1. *Non-soaking:* Start cooking the grain very slowly over a low flame, in an uncovered pressure cooker. Do not put any salt in yet so that it will take more time to come to a boil. When it comes to a boil, add the salt, cover, and bring up to pressure (it is up when the gauge hisses). Then, place a heat deflector underneath (make sure the flame is on medium-low) and simmer for 45 to 50 minutes.

2. *Soaking:* Soak the rice (covered with cold water) for 3 to 5 hours or overnight. Place in the pressure cooker (along with the soaking water). This time, add salt and cover right away (otherwise it may turn out too soggy). Put on a medium-high flame and bring up to pressure. When it is up, turn the flame down to medium-low, place a heat deflector underneath, and simmer for 45 to 50 minutes.

A note about salt: In some of the following recipes there is a general amount of salt listed in the ingredients: one to three pinches of sea salt. As sea salt is a very yang combination of minerals, persons with more yang conditions can use less, (stress and/or hypertension from a yang cause), while those with a more yin condition can use a little more—three pinches is plenty. Those who are experiencing stress and/or hypertension from both extremes can use a middle amount.

Some dishes, like rice with beans, rice with lotus seeds, or rice with seeds require a little more salt to make them more digestible, so a larger amount is indicated as minimum (2 to 3 pinches of sea salt).

Basic Brown Rice (Pressure-Cooked)
(Use every day, the principal food for all conditions.)

3 cups brown rice
3¾–4½ cups spring water
3 pinches sea salt

Pressure-cook following one of the above methods. Let the pressure come down completely before removing the cover. Scoop out the rice, with a wet rice paddle or wooden spoon, into a wooden bowl as you separate and air out the lumps.

The bottom rice can be mixed in if it is not burnt. Keep the brown side turned down and totally covered to help keep it soft. If the bottom is really stuck to the pot, keep a 1-inch layer of rice in the pot, put the lid back on, and let it sit for 20 to 30 minutes. The warmth of the fresh rice will help to loosen and soften the bottom.

Keep the rice covered with a bamboo or sushi mat. This will protect it while letting air circulate. When ready to serve, dish the rice into individual bowls. Serves 6.

Azuki Bean Rice
(Helps strengthen the kidneys and adrenals.)

> $2\frac{1}{2}$ cups brown rice, washed
> $\frac{1}{2}$ cup azuki beans, washed
> $4\frac{1}{2}$ cups spring water
> 2 pinches sea salt
> 1 piece kombu, $1\frac{1}{2}$" long

Boil azuki beans with the kombu in 2 cups of water for 10 to 15 minutes until the water becomes red. Cool the beans until they are lukewarm. Put the rice in the pressure cooker with the beans and their red, boiled juice. Use pressure-cooking method #1 (*Non-soaking*) and follow the directions for *Basic Brown Rice*. Or, soak the rice and beans together overnight and use method #2 (*Soaking*). Serves 6.

Lotus Seed Rice
(The addition of lotus seeds makes this dish especially strengthening for the lungs and the kidneys.)

> $2\frac{1}{2}$ cups rice
> $\frac{1}{2}$ cup lotus seeds
> $4\frac{1}{2}$ cups spring water
> 3 pinches sea salt

Wash and soak lotus seeds and rice 3 to 4 hours or overnight. Pressure-cook using method #2 and following the directions for *Basic Brown Rice* (*Pressure-cooked*). Serves 6.

Sesame Seed Rice
(Helps improve general vitality.)

> $2\frac{1}{2}$ cups brown rice
> $\frac{1}{2}$ cup roasted white or black sesame seeds
> $3 \frac{3}{4}$–$4\frac{1}{2}$ cups spring water
> 3 pinches sea salt

Wash and quickly roast the sesame seeds, being careful not to burn them. Stir the seeds constantly with a wooden spoon until a nutty fragrance is emitted. Combine with all the other ingredients and cook as in *Basic Brown Rice* (*Pressure-cooked*). Serves 6.

Sweet Rice and Millet
(Strengthens spleen, pancreas, and stomach.)

 2 cups sweet rice
 1 cup millet
 4 cups spring water
 3 pinches sea salt

Wash and combine all the ingredients and cook as in *Basic Brown Rice* (*Pressure-cooked*), method #2 (minus the soaking) for 40 to 45 minutes. Serves 6.

Rice with Kombu
(This dish is helpful for more yang persons who have taken too much salt.)

 3 cups rice
 4–4½ cups spring water
 1 strip kombu, 1″

Wash and cook rice as in *Basic Brown Rice* (either method), using kombu instead of sea salt.

Rice with Pearl Barley
(This dish is helpful for dissolving hardened fats and animal foods and especially good for those with a more yang condition.)

 2½ cups brown rice
 ½ cup pearl barley
 4–4½ cups water
 1–3 pinches sea salt

Wash rice and barley, mix, and cook as in *Basic Brown Rice* (either method).

Variations:
   1. Barley Rice: 2½ cups rice with ½ cup whole barley. Use method #2 as barley needs to be soaked.
   2. Millet Rice: 2 cups rice and 1 cup millet
   3. Rice with Sweet Rice: 2 cups rice and 1 cup sweet rice

4. Rice with Wheat Berries: 2½ to 2¾ cups rice and ¼ to ½ cup wheat berries. Use method #2 as wheat berries need soaking.

5. Rice, Sweet Rice, and Rye: 2 cups rice, ¾ cup sweet rice, and ½ cup rye berries. Method #2.

6. Chick-pea Rice: 2½ cups rice and ½ cup chick-peas. Method #2.

7. Rice with Chick-peas and Wheat Berries: 2 cups rice, ½ cup chick-peas, and ½ cup wheat berries. Method #2.

8. Azuki Sweet Rice or Black Soybean Sweet Rice: 2½ cups sweet rice and ¼ cup azuki beans or black soybeans. Method #2.

9. Soybean Rice: 2½ cups rice with ½ cup black or yellow soybeans. Beans can be roasted or soaked overnight.

10. Rice with Wild Rice: 2½ cups rice with ½ cup wild rice

11. Chestnut Rice: 2 cups rice and 1 cup dried chestnuts. You can also make rice, sweet rice, and chestnuts.

12. Rice with Fresh Corn: 2 cups rice, 1 cup fresh corn kernels, and 3 cups of water. For a lighter variation, make *Basic Brown Rice* and mix in cooked corn kernels after the rice is cooked.

13. Rice with Squash: 2½ cups rice and 1 cup diced winter squash.

14. Umeboshi Rice: 3 cups brown rice and 1 umeboshi plum instead of sea salt.

15. Bancha Rice: Use bancha tea instead of water.

16. Scallion Rice: *Basic Brown Rice* with 1 cup finely chopped scallions mixed in as you take the hot rice out of the pressure cooker.

17. Brown Rice with Shiso Leaves: *Basic Brown Rice* with ⅓ cup shiso leaves (finely chopped) mixed in as you take the rice out of the pressure cooker.

18. Rice with Sunflower Seeds or Pumpkin Seeds: Toasted seeds can be pressure-cooked with rice or mixed in to hot rice as you take it out of the pressure cooker.

19. Almond Rice: *Basic Brown Rice* with ⅔ cup almonds which have been blanched, skinned, and chopped. You can add chopped parsley, scallions, or chives after cooking.

Basic Brown Rice (Boiled)

2 cups brown rice, washed
4 cups spring water

2 pinches sea salt

Put washed rice into a pot (preferably with a heavy lid) with water and salt. Bring to a boil, then lower the flame, place a heat deflector underneath, and simmer for about 1 hour or until all the water has been absorbed. Wet a wooden spoon or rice paddle and dish out the rice into a wooden bowl. Cover with a sushi or bamboo mat. Serves 4.

Variations:

1. . **Roasted Boiled Rice:** Toast grain in a dry skillet, stirring constantly, until it is slightly golden and has a nutty aroma. Bring water to a boil, add rice and salt and proceed according to *Basic Brown Rice (Boiled)*. This makes the rice more digestible and gives it a lighter, fluffier texture.
2. **Soaked Boiled Rice:** Soak rice overnight and proceed according to recipe. This also will help make rice more digestible. Rice can also be roasted, then soaked and boiled.
3. **Boiled Long-Grain Rice:** Substitute long-grain rice for short or medium grain.
4. **Rice Pilaf:** Toast rice as above. When rice is almost done, add ¼ cup each of finely chopped onions, celery, and carrots. Roast with grain until grain is done, then proceed as in *Basic Brown Rice (Boiled)*.

Many of the variations in *Basic Brown Rice (Pressure-cooked)* can also be applied to boiled rice. Millet Rice, Barley Rice (roast barley and soak overnight), Rice with Shiso Leaves, Scallion Rice, and Rice with Wild Rice, are examples.

Soft Rice (Plain)

1 cup brown rice
5 cups water
1 pinch sea salt

Cook as in *Basic Brown Rice (Pressure-cooked)*. Soft rice can also be prepared by simmering it overnight over a low flame and a heat deflector. In this case, use 10 cups of water to every cup of rice. Serves 5.

Ojiya (Soft Rice with Miso)

2 cups leftover cooked brown rice
4–5 cups spring water

2 level tsps. miso
1 strip kombu, 1½" long, washed, soaked, and sliced
3–4 sliced scallions

Place the kombu on the bottom of a pot or pressure cooker. Add the rice and water and bring them to a boil or up to pressure. Turn the flame to low, place a deflector underneath, and simmer or pressure-cook for ½ hour. Add 1 tablespoon or so of water to the miso and stir it in until the miso becomes a purée. Uncover the rice (wait until the pressure is down if using a pressure cooker), and then put it back onto the stove. Mix in the miso, simmer for another 3 to 5 minutes, then turn off the flame. Garnish with sliced scallions and serve immediately. Serves 4 to 5.

Rice Cream with Nori and Umeboshi
(Rice cream is a dish with special healing qualities. It helps purify blood and lymph.)

1 cup dry-roasted brown rice
3–6 cups spring water
1 pinch sea salt
1 sheet toasted nori
1 umeboshi plum
Cheesecloth

Pressure-cook with salt and water for 1 hour following directions for *Basic Brown Rice* (*Pressure-cooked*). Make a sack out of clean cheesecloth. Cool off the cooked rice, place some inside the sack and squeeze out as much of the creamy liquid as you can. Reheat and serve with nori and an umeboshi plum. The leftover pulp can be eaten separately or added to soup or vegetable dishes.

Especially good condiments for this dish are gomashio, umeboshi, toasted nori, green nori flakes, tekka, and shiso leaves. Serves 2.

Musubi (Rice Ball)
(Great for lunches, picnics, and trips, rice balls are also a very strengthening, stabilizing way to eat rice.)

1 cup cooked short-grain (sticks well) brown rice
2 quarters of a nori sheet (a sheet cut in half then half again)
1 pinch sea salt
1 umeboshi plum (or ½ if it is large)

Toast nori by passing it over an open flame a few times, until it becomes green but not so much that it becomes crisp and crinkly. Tear it into 4 pieces.

Wet hands (to prevent the rice from sticking to them) in a bowl of salted water. While holding the rice, stick an umeboshi plum in the middle (the pit may be removed if desired). Tightly mold the rice around the plum in an English-muffin shape or a flat triangle and put it on a plate.

With dry hands, use a quarter sheet of nori (the shiny side on the outside), to cover each side of the rice ball. Firmly mold it on. The rice ball is now ready to eat, or pack it up and take it on a trip to consume later. Serves 1.

Basic Fried Rice

4 cups cooked short-grain brown rice
Kernels from 4 ears of corn, cooked
1 onion, sliced in thin half-moons
1 Tbsp. dark (toasted) sesame oil or a small amount of spring water
Tamari soy sauce

Sauté the onion in a skillet a few minutes, being careful not to let it burn. Add rice, layering it over the onion. Cover the skillet, and cook approximately 15 minutes, adding a little water to prevent burning. Add the corn and a sprinkling of tamari soy sauce, mix well, and cook 5 to 10 minutes more. Garnish with chopped scallions or parsley. Serves 3 to 4.

Variations: Other vegetables, like carrots, cabbage, fresh corn, and minced scallion roots, as well as fresh tofu, and cooked tempeh or seitan can be added to fried rice. You can cook them with or just after the onions are added.

Rice Salad
(This is a nice summer dish.)

3 cups cooked rice
$\frac{1}{2}$ cup diced carrots, lightly cooked
$\frac{1}{2}$ cup fresh peas, lightly cooked
$\frac{1}{2}$ cup fresh corn kernels, lightly cooked
1 Tbsp. sweet rice vinegar and 1 tsp. tamari soy sauce
or
1 Tbsp. umeboshi vinegar

Mix together rice and vegetables. Mix vinegar and tamari soy sauce and toss with salad. (Just mix in umeboshi vinegar if you choose that.) Garnish with sprigs of parsley.

Variations: Other vegetables can be added or substituted. Broccoli flowerets, celery, burdock, lotus root, pickles, sauerkraut, or snow peas are some examples. Cooked beans, tempeh, or seitan can also be used. Finely chopped scallions, parsley, or celery leaves can be added. Small, cooked shrimp with rice salad is another variation. Dressings can be made with lemon juice and tamari soy sauce, or with grated ginger juice for more options.

Mochi (Homemade)

4 cups sweet rice
4 cups water
4 pinches sea salt
A handful of sweet rice flour (optional)

Cook as in *Basic Brown Rice* (*Pressure-cooked*). When done, in a wooden bowl, vigorously pound the rice with a large wooden pestle (which is moistened initially and from time to time to prevent the rice from sticking to it) until all the grains are crushed and form a smooth, sticky mass. This may take a half hour. Sprinkle some flour onto a baking sheet and layer the rice on top (up to 1-inch thick). Dry this for 1 to 2 days and then store it in the refrigerator.

To serve, cut the mochi into small pieces and toast them in a skillet with or without oil until they become soft. This only takes a few minutes. (Turn them over when they are half done so that both sides toast evenly.) Serve them with some raw grated daikon with a few drops of tamari soy sauce added. The daikon helps in digestion of the mochi. Serves 5 to 6.

Fortunately, mochi can now be purchased in some natural food stores. In this case, all that is needed is to toast it for a few minutes in the oven or in a dry frying pan over a medium-low flame to avoid burning.

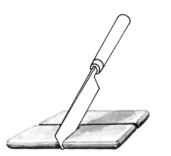

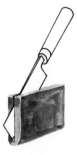

Fig. 6 Mochi

Millet:————————————————————————————

Millet is a more yang grain, being small, round, and more alkaline. It is good for the spleen and pancreas, it helps to settle an acidic stomach, and it gives warmth. For helping to relieve blood glucose disorders millet can be considered as a major grain after rice.

Millet cooks fairly quickly and comes out very soft, so it can, but does not need to be pressure-cooked. It can also be cooked in combination with rice, using 10 to 15 percent millet. Millet can be made either light and fluffy, or moist and creamy like a porridge. The fluffy style can be a little dry, so it can often be eaten with a sauce or cooked with other ingredients. A standard combination uses squash. Other common companions are vegetables like carrots and onions as well as roasted seeds.

Millet (Dry)

1 cup millet, washed
2 cups spring water
1 pinch sea salt

Bring the salt and water to a boil and slowly and carefully add the millet. Let this come to a boil again. Then, cover the pot, turn the flame to medium-low, place a heat deflector underneath, and simmer for about 30 minutes. Serves 2.

Variations:

1. Toasted, Boiled Millet: Millet can be dry-roasted before boiling. To do this, heat a skillet on medium heat. Wash millet and add to pan. Stir constantly until millet is slightly golden and has a delicious nutty aroma. Cook as in the recipe for *Fluffy Millet*. Millet can also be toasted with a small amount of sesame oil.
2. Millet with Vegetables: Many vegetables, like winter squash, carrots, onions, leeks, corn on the cob, celery, and burdock, can be boiled with millet. (Millet can be toasted or not.) Cooked seitan can also be cooked with millet.
3. Millet with Scallions: Fresh, finely chopped scallions or parsley can be added to millet at the end of cooking. Occasionally, toasted seeds can also be added at the end of cooking.
4. Millet with Sauce: Millet can be cooked in any of the mentioned methods and served with a light kuzu sauce. (See *Sauces and Dressings* chapter.) A nice combination might be

millet, roasted and then cooked with diced onions, carrots, and corn off the cob. A little fresh, chopped parsley can be mixed in at the end of cooking and millet can be served with a light kuzu sauce with a little scallions mixed in.

Millet Porridge

1 cup millet, washed
4 cups boiling water
1 pinch sea salt

Bring salt and water to a boil. Carefully pour the millet into the pot of boiling water. Bring to a boil again, turn the flame to low, place a heat deflector underneath, cover, and simmer for 30 minutes. Serves 3.

Millet and Squash

2 cups millet
1 small winter squash
2½ cups spring water
2 pinches sea salt

Wash millet and dry-roast in a skillet approximately 5 to 8 minutes, or until lightly browned. Place the millet and squash in a pressure cooker with water and salt, and pressure-cook 25 minutes. Bring pressure down immediately. Serves 4.

Variations:
   1.   **Millet and Cauliflower:** 1 cup millet, 1 cup cauliflower, and up to 3½ cups water.
   2.   **Millet, Squash, and Onions:** 1 cup millet, ½ cup winter squash, and ½ cup onions.
   3.   **Pressure-cooked Millet:** Follow the recipe for *Millet and Squash*, except reduce water to 2 cups. Pressure-cook for 15 to 20 minutes.
   4.   **Other variations:** Many of the variations for *Fluffy Millet* can also be applied to this recipe. Millet can also be pureed in a food mill (a hand-powered food mill), and served with a light kuzu sauce.

Pressure-cooked Millet Gomoku

2 cups millet	**½ cup diced onions**
2–3 ears of corn off the cob	**½ cup diced, cooked seitan**
½ cup diced carrots	**3 cups spring water**
¼ cup diced burdock	**Chopped parsley for garnish**

¹/₂ cup diced celery

Wash, then dry-roast millet until golden brown. Put millet, vegetables, and seitan in a pressure cooker. Add water. (Salt is not necessary as there is tamari soy sauce in the seitan.) Secure pressure-cooker lid and place over a medium-high flame. Bring up to pressure, reduce heat to medium-low, and place a flame deflector under pot. Cook for 15 minutes. Remove the pot from heat and let pressure come down by itself. Remove cover and transfer millet to serving bowl. Garnish with chopped parsley and serve.

Variations:
   1. Millet Croquettes: After millet is cooked and parsley is added, allow it to cool until it is easy to handle. Shape millet into croquettes and serve as is, or lightly brown it in a skillet with or without a little oil. This can also be served with a light kuzu, ginger sauce.
   2. Millet Loaf: After cooking, millet can be pressed into a bread pan while it is still hot. Let cool almost to room temperature. Millet will adhere to itself and hold its shape when cut. This can be served as is, with a chopped parsley garnish, or a light kuzu sauce.

Barley

Barley is delicious and light and has a cooling and calming energy. (This is particularly helpful for people with a more yang condition.) There are basically two types of barley:

Hulled barley: Hulled barley is the whole barley grain with the husk removed. It is mild tasting and nourishing and requires a little more preparation than either rice or millet. Whole barley is most often soaked, then pressure-cooked or boiled. It can be made as a grain dish by itself, cooked with rice, or used in soups, stews, and salads.
   Pearled and polished barley are refined versions of this grain. Although you could use either on occasion, whole barley is preferred as a staple grain.

Pearl barley: Pearl barley is actually a grass rather than a grain. Also known as Jobs' Tears, it has qualities similar to whole barley but is much more yin. Pearl barley is also known for its ability to break down hardened animal fats within the body. It is not usually eaten alone, and is often cooked with rice. It can also be used in making soups and stews.

Pearl barley is very helpful for persons with a more yang condition, but because of its more yin qualities, those with a more yin condition can use it infrequently or avoid it altogether.

Pressure-cooked Barley

1 cup whole barley
1½–2 cups water
1 pinch sea salt

Wash barley as you would rice. Soak for at least 4 hours in 1½ to 2 cups water. (It can be soaked overnight.) Place in a pressure cooker with sea salt and cook as in *Basic Brown Rice (Pressure-cooked)*.

Variations:

Barley with Seitan and Vegetables: Pressure-cook the following with barley: ½ cup diced seitan, ½ cup diced carrot, and ¼ cup diced shiitake, and add ½ cup chopped parsley when you take barley out of the pressure cooker.
Barley with Kombu: Barley can be cooked with 1 to 3 inches of kombu instead of sea salt. (You can also use kombu and sea salt together for a heartier dish.)
Other variations: By adding umeboshi vinegar to cooked, cooled barley (either plain or with other ingredients), you can make a barley salad. Leftover barley can also be fried as you would rice.

Soft Barley

1 cup barley
4–5 cups spring water
1 pinch sea salt
Several parsley sprigs

Boil as in *Basic Brown Rice (Boiled)*. Simmer for 1¼ to 1½ hours or until soft. Garnish with the parsley. Serves 5.

Variations:
Barley Cereal can also be made with kombu and or vegetables. An alternate way of cooking is to bring unsoaked barley, water, and sea salt to a boil, cover, and put on a very

low flame on a flame tamer. Cook overnight. In the morning
you will have ready-made hot cereal. (This is especially good
in the cooler months of the year.) Try barley with winter
squash and kombu cooked this way.

Pearl Barley Rice: See *Rice with Pearl Barley* under *Basic
Brown Rice* variations. This can also be made into breakfast
cereal by using more water.

Buckwheat:

Buckwheat can grow in a very cold climate and has a short growing
season. This grain gives strength, generates heat, and is good for the
lungs, kidneys, and bladder. It is particularly appropriate as a winter
food but should be used only occasionally by persons who are ill.
Persons who have had surgery within a year's time should avoid
using buckwheat at all for several months.

Buckwheat can be cooked just like millet as it also cooks quickly
and is a very soft grain.

Kasha

1 cup buckwheat groats   Chopped scallions or
2 cups boiling spring water   parsley for garnish
1 pinch sea salt

Wash buckwheat and dry-roast in a frying pan for several
minutes. Put the grain in a pot and add the boiling water and
salt. Bring to a boil, lower the heat and simmer for 20 to
30 minutes, or until the water has been absorbed. Garnish with
chopped scallions or parsley and serve.

Variations: Cook buckwheat with sautéed cabbage and carrots, (for those with a more yin condition), or cook with
onions, adding chopped parsley at the end. Buckwheat can
also be fried like rice and garnished with plenty of chopped
scallions. (For more yin conditions, mostly eaten in winter.)

Creamy Kasha

1 cup buckwheat groats
2 scallions
5 cups spring water
1 pinch sea salt

Wash the buckwheat and put it into a pot. Add cold water

and sea salt and bring to a boil. Then turn the flame down to low, place a flame deflector underneath, and cook for 20 to 30 minutes. Wash and slice the scallions for a garnish. Serves 3.

Buckwheat Salad

1 cup buckwheat groats
½ cup chopped, drained sauerkraut (save liquid)
1 cup steamed, chopped kale
2 Tbsps. finely chopped parsley
2 cups spring water plus the sauerkraut juice
Pinch sea salt

Wash the buckwheat and dry-roast it for several minutes in a frying pan. Bring the water and the drained sauerkraut juice to a boil. Add the buckwheat and salt to the boiling liquid. Cover and cook for 20 minutes.

Sauté finely chopped parsley in a very small amount of water. Mix the parsley, kale, and sauerkraut with buckwheat. Add dressing described below.

Dressing: 2 Tbsps. tamari soy sauce and 1 tsp. fresh squeezed ginger juice

Variation: Add sautéed or fried tempeh and cook with buckwheat.

Oats:

Oats have more protein and fat than other grains. Therefore, while they are helpful to produce more warmth in the body, they should not be taken on a daily basis as they can cause a buildup of mucus. Use about two times a week maximum during the initial healing stage, and use whole oats whenever possible.

Whole Oatmeal

1 cup whole oats, washed
5–6 cups spring water
1″-strip of kombu

Soak the oats for several hours or overnight. Put them in a pot, add the water and kombu, cover, and bring to a boil. Reduce the heat and simmer over a low heat for several hours, or overnight, until water is absorbed. Use a flame deflector to prevent burning. Dulse flakes, sea vegetable powders, or gomashio make a nice garnish.

Scotch Oats

> 1 cup Scotch oats
> 3 cups water
> 1 pinch sea salt
> 1 strip kombu, 2"–4"

Combine water, salt, and kombu, and bring to a boil. Wash and dry-roast oats in a skillet for 5 minutes, stirring with a wooden spoon over a medium-low flame. Then, carefully pour oats into the boiling water. Bring back to a boil, turn heat to medium-low, place a flame deflector underneath, and cook for about 30 to 40 minutes. Serves 2.

Variations: Both whole oats and Scotch oats can be cooked with vegetables. (Try whole oats cooked overnight with onions.) Oats can also be cooked without kombu, and you can cook them with dulse as an alternative. (Whole oats pressure-cooked with onions, carrots, celery, and dulse makes a nice porridge.) On occasion, persons with a more yang condition could cook oats with raisins for a sweet breakfast cereal. Oats can be garnished with chopped scallions, parsley, toasted nori, sometimes roasted seeds, and/or a favorite condiment (gomashio, shiso leaf powder, etc.).

Oatmeal (Rolled Oats)

> 1 cup rolled oats
> 3 cups water
> 1 pinch sea salt
> Optional: 1 strip kombu, 2"–4", kombu, soaked 20 minutes

If using kombu, cut it into ½-inch pieces. Bring water to a boil, including kombu soaking water. Add salt and oats. (They can be toasted or not.) Reduce heat to medium-low, place a flame deflector underneath, and simmer for 20 minutes or more.

The same variations for whole oats and Scotch oats apply here. Corn off the cob and celery cooked with oats makes a nice addition for a summer breakfast.

Wheat: ———————————————————————

Wheat berries are harder to digest than other grains. They should always be soaked beforehand. Make sure you chew really well in order to insure good digestion.

Pressure-cook like rice except that the wheat berries need to be soaked for several hours or overnight. You may also need to cook them an extra 10 to 15 minutes. Use twice as much water as grain.

Wheat also comes in the form of bulgur, which has been partially boiled, dried, and then ground; and couscous, which has been refined and cracked. Both of these wheat products are convenient, as they cook very quickly, especially couscous. However, they should not be used as staple foods since a great deal of nutrition is lost in their processing. Use them as an occasional treat and for variety.

Azuki Bean Wheat Berries

2 cups wheat berries
½–¾ cup azuki beans
4–5 cups spring water
2 pinches sea salt

Wash and soak wheat berries and beans together for 3 to 5 hours or overnight. Pressure-cook as in *Basic Brown Rice*. Simmer for 60 to 70 minutes. Serves 6 to 8.

Bulgur and Vegetables

1 cup bulghur
¼ cup each diced onions, carrots, and celery
2–2¼ cups spring water
1 pinch sea salt

Bring salt and water to a boil. Meanwhile, wash and dice the vegetables and layer them (onions on the bottom, then celery, and finally carrots on top) in another pot. Add some water (just enough to cover the vegetables) and simmer until they are soft. Then, add the bulgur, pour the boiling water on top, cover, and bring to a boil again. Turn the flame to low and simmer for 20 minutes. Serves 3.

Boiled Couscous

1 cup couscous
2½ cups spring water
1 pinch sea salt
Optional: **1 tsp. sesame oil**

Bring the water, salt, and optional oil to a boil. Pour in the couscous, turn the flame to low, cover, and simmer for 5 minutes. Add some garnish or sauce. Serves 2.

Variations: Couscous with vegetables can be made by simmering vegetables in kombu stock until tender before adding couscous. Cooked chick-peas, seitan, or fish can be added with vegetables for a heartier dish. Cooked couscous can be molded or shaped into croquettes. Tamari soy sauce or miso can be added as seasoning.

Rye:

Rye is a harder grain like wheat and is most often used as flour in breads, crackers, or other baked products. It requires longer cooking than most other grains and is very chewy. (Chew very well.) Rye is used in its whole form to make some unique and delicious dishes.

Basic Rye

2 cups rye
$2\frac{1}{2}$–3 cups water
2 pinches sea salt

Cook in the same way as for *Basic Brown Rice* (*Pressure-cooked*), and use the soaking method. (Soak rye overnight.)

Rye and Vegetables

2 cups rye
5 cups water
1 cup diced carrots
1 medium-sized onion, diced
1 ear fresh corn
1 bunch parsley or watercress
1 umeboshi plum
Sea salt
Optional: 1 Tbsp. grated ginger root

Wash and dry-roast rye in a frying pan for about 5 minutes. Put the roasted rye in a pressure cooker, add 2 cups water, and pressure-cook for 45 minutes. Boil the carrots, onion, and corn on the cob for 1 minute with 2 pinches of sea salt. Dip the parsley or watercress into a saucepan of boiling water for 1 minute. (Do not use salted water for this as the greens will become bitter.)

Drain and chop the parsley or watercress. Scrape the kernels from the corn cob and add them to the rye in the pressure cooker. Add the onions and carrots, and place the greens on top. Dissolve 1 sliced umeboshi in a little water and add it to the grain and vegetables. Grated ginger root may also be added for flavoring. Mix well and serve as a salad in a large bowl.

Corn:

The corn eaten by the native American Indians was much hardier, stronger, smaller, and nutritious than most of the commercial corn available today. This grain was more effective in maintaining one's health, particularly strengthening the heart and blood vessels.

During the healing stage use only corn dishes that have been cooked whole at the beginning, such as whole corn dishes and traditional *masa, tortillas,* and so on. Avoid dishes that have been ground previous to any cooking, as they may cause a buildup of mucus.

There are five main types of corn available today:
1. *Sweet corn*—The regular corn on the cob.
2. *Dent corn*—Corn with dented kernels used for making cornmeal.
3. *Flour corn*—Starchy variety used in Latin American cooking.
4. *Flint corn*—Starchy variety used in Latin America Cooking.
5. *Popcorn.*

Fig. 7 Corn

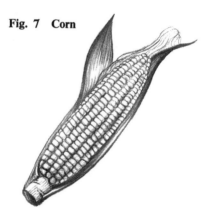

Corn on the Cob (Boiled)

Desired number of ears of fresh corn
A large pot of water
Umeboshi paste

Trim away the dry, outer leaves of the corn, but keep the fresher inner wrapping intact. Chop off the excess straggly husk ends and silk hairs on the top end of the corn. Put sea salt in the water and bring the pot to a boil. Drop the corn in and boil for about 10 minutes. Take out the corn and serve. After unhusking individual ears of corn, umeboshi paste can be rubbed on it if desired. Strain out any leftover silk hairs in the liquid with an oil skimmer and use this liquid for soup stock.

Dried Whole Corn (Dent)

2 cups whole, dried dent corn
8 cups spring water
2 pinches sea salt
1 cup sifted wood ash

Wash and soak the corn overnight. Put the corn, 4 cups of water, and the wood ash (no salt) in a pressure cooker. Cook for 30 to 45 minutes. When the corn is done, put it into a colander or strainer. Rinse out all the ash and remove the corn skins. (If the skins are not loose enough, cook again with more ashes for another 10 minutes.) Pressure-cook the un-hulled corn for 1 hour in a clean pot with salt and 4 more cups of water. The corn can be served as it is, or used as a base for other corn recipes (see below). Serves 4 to 6.

Masa (Corn Dough)

4 cups whole, dried flint corn
8–10 cups water initially and 8 more cups later
1 cup sifted wood ash
3–4 pinches sea salt

Follow the directions in *Dried Whole Corn* but use 8 to 10 cups of water in the beginning and 8 more cups after the corn is hulled. Take out and cool the corn. Grind it in a hand grinder (not a blender). Knead this for about 15 minutes. Moisten it with a little water if it is too dry. If not using the dough immediately, store it in the refrigerator (up to a week). This is the base for many corn recipes such as arepas, tortillas, cereals, and so on.

Arepas

3 cups masa corn dough (see above recipe)
Boiling water
Water to help shape the dough
2–3 pinches sea salt
1 Tbsp. sesame oil
Optional: $\frac{1}{2}$ cup roasted sesame seeds

Knead the dough while mixing in salt and optional sesame

seeds. It should feel like bread dough. If it is too dry, add a little water, and if too wet, add more dough or let it sit and dry for a few minutes. Separate it into balls which are molded into English-muffin shapes, except a little flatter. Boil some water, put the balls in, and remove them when they rise to the top.

Heat some oil in a skillet, place the arepas inside, cover, and cook them over a low flame for about 15 to 20 minutes. (Turn them over halfway through to cook the other side.) If desired, this is the time to slit them open and stuff them with beans and/or vegetables. Serves 4 to 6.

Tortillas

Follow the method described in Arepas, except after you have kneaded the dough, form into 1½-inch balls. Place a ball between 2 layers of wax paper or plastic wrap. Roll out to a ¼-inch thickness with a rolling pin. Heat a skillet on medium-low heat. (Cast iron works best.) Cook tortillas, one at a time, browning on each side (about 8 to 10 minutes total).

Tortillas can be served as is or rolled up with beans, seitan, scrambled tofu, and/or vegetables. Leftover azuki-squash dish with fresh chopped scallions makes a delicious filling.

Grain Products:———————————————————————————

During the initial healing period it is better to avoid flour or refined-grain products altogether. This is particularly so for any dry, roasted, or baked items such as bread, crackers, granola, and others. However, boiled, whole-grain flour products may be used occasionally for variety, including noodles, fu, and seitan. Remember however, it may be necessary·to avoid buckwheat noodles in some cases for a period of time.

1. Noodles are a great snack and cook up very quickly. There are several types which are now available in most natural food stores.

    A. *Soba*—Long, thin, Oriental buckwheat noodles.
        1) Buckwheat with/without wheat in varying amounts
        2) Jinenjo soba (contains jinenjo flour)
        3) *Ito* soba—Extra thin and light
        4) Buckwheat *ramen*—Instant buckwheat noodles
    B. *Udon*—Long, Oriental whole wheat noodles.

1) Thicker than soba and contains wholewheat and sometimes unbleached, sifted white flour
2) *Somen*—Very thin wheat noodles
3) Ramen—Instant noodles

C. *Pasta*—Wheat alone or in combination with other grain
flours.
1) Spaghetti
2) Shells
3) Spirals
4) Elbows
5) Ribbons
6) Ziti
7) Rigatoni
8) Linguini
9) Lasagna
10) Alphabets, etc.

Buy these noodles, especially the ramen and pasta, from natural
food stores. The ramen bought in Oriental shops may contain
animal fats, sugar, MSG, chemicals, additives, and food coloring.
Pasta bought in a regular store usually contain eggs which are
best avoided.

To cook noodles, place them in a large pot of boiling water. (Too
little water causes them to clump together.) As the pasta is added, stir
and separate the noodles with a long chopstick to prevent them from
lying side by side in a parallel fashion, otherwise they will stick together. (This precaution is basically for long thin noodles such as
udon and soba.)

Keep the flame high and add a little cold water each time the pot
comes to a boil, until the noodles are soft (usually about 3 times). Or,
turn the flame down a bit after adding the noodles, and simmer until
they are cooked. The first method is preferred as the noodles come
out more firm and crisp. When done, the inside is the same color as
the outside. Drain them in a colander and immediately run cold
water over them. This helps to keep them from clumping together.

Avoid making noodles too soggy, especially if they are later going
to be reheated or fried. Pay special attention to the somen and Ito
soba, as they cook up very quickly and are absolutely horrible when
soft and mushy.

Add a pinch of salt when boiling pasta. (Udon and soba already
contain salt so they don't need it.) The leftover noodle water can be
used in soup stocks.

Noodles in Broth

1 pack udon or soba noodles previously boiled
1 1" to 2" piece kombu
1 shiitake mushroom, soaked and sliced
4 cups spring water, including shiitake soaking water
½ cake tofu, cut into small cubes
3 Tbsps. tamari soy sauce
1–2 sheets toasted nori, cut into small pieces
3 chopped scallions

Make a soup stock by bringing kombu, shiitake, and water to a boil, and simmering for 5 minutes. Take out the kombu and shiitake. Boil the tofu cubes and take them out when they rise to the top. Add the tamari and simmer for 5 to 7 minutes. Put in some noodles (only add what you are immediately going to eat and keep the rest aside) until they become warm, then dish them out into individual bowls. Place some tofu, shiitake slices, nori, and scallions on top of each bowl, pour some broth over them and serve.

For variation:

1) Add different kinds of sea vegetables, root, or green vegetables into the broth, boil them until soft, and add the tamari soy sauce.
2) Add different kinds of sea vegetables, and/or boiled, sautéed, or thinly sliced raw vegetables as a garnish. Roasted seeds, fu (soak and boil it in the broth previously, as was done with the tofu above), cooked seitan and tempeh, and grated daikon or ginger can also be added.
3) As a general rule, anything can be added as long as there is a sea vegetable in the broth, and a pungent item in the garnish. This would include scallions, diced cooked onions, chives, or daikon, as they help digestion.

Zaru Soba

Soba, previously boiled
1 Tbsp. tamari soy sauce
1 Tbsp. brown rice vinegar
4 Tbsps. kombu soup stock
Chopped scallions
Nori, toasted and cut into thin strips

Place soba noodles onto an individual serving plate and place a few strips of nori on top. (In Japan they have special individual bamboo serving "plates" which allows soba to drain.) Combine tamari soy sauce, rice vinegar, kombu stock, and scallions into a small bowl to make a dip for the noodles. Make a dip for each person.

Noodle Salad

8 oz. noodles of choice, cooked
2 carrots
1½ cup broccoli flowerets
½ cup sliced green beans
¼ cup finely chopped scallions
Favorite tofu dressing (see chapter on Dressings)

Wash carrots and cut to desired shape. Bring a pot of water to a boil. Add a pinch of sea salt. Add carrots and cook until done all the way through, but still crunchy. Remove from water and drain. Cook the green beans in the same manner, and then the broccoli. Mix vegetables, noodles, and scallions. Place in a large bowl and serve with tofu dressing poured on top, or on the side.

Noodles with Carrot Miso Sauce

8 oz. pkg. udon or whole wheat spaghetti
1 recipe of *Carrot Miso Sauce*
½ cup chopped scallions

Cook noodles as described in the beginning of this section. Rinse and drain. Make *Carrot Miso Sauce*. Place noodles on an attractive serving dish and pour hot sauce over the top. Garnish with chopped scallions.

Fried Noodles (Water-Sautéed)

4 cups spring water
1 package soba or udon noodles
2 cups shredded cabbage
1–2 Tbsps. tamari soy sauce
½ cup sliced scallions

Boil the noodles, rinse them under cold water, and drain. Place a small amount of spring water in a frying pan and add the cabbage. Put the cooked noodles on top of the cabbage, cover the pan, and cook over low heat for 5 to 7 minutes, or until the noodles are warm. Add the tamari soy sauce and mix the noodles and vegetables well. Do not stir the ingredients together until this time; they should be left to cook peacefully until the very end. Cook for several minutes longer and add the scallions at the very end. Serve hot or cold.

Variations: Any kind of vegetable can be used in fried noodles. Cooked tofu, seitan, fu, dried tofu, or tempeh can also be added. Toasted sesame seeds and toasted nori strips can also be used for a garnish, along with ginger or scallions. (You need to add either ginger or scallion as they will help you digest the oil.)

2. Seitan is a protein-rich wheat product. It is made from the gluten of hard spring or winter wheat flours.

Seitan

(Seitan can also be bought in natural food stores. Avoid ones that have been heavily spiced if in the process of healing.)

3½ lbs. whole wheat flour (spring or winter)
8–9 cups of water

Place the flour into a large stainless-steel mixing bowl, and gradually add the water. Form a dough and knead it for 5 to 15 minutes until it becomes stiff and earlobe consistency.

Submerge the dough in water and let it sit for 5 to 10 minutes. Then knead and separate the dough in the water until the liquid is full of bran and starch.

Drain the seitan in a colander which is placed inside a large pot. (If desired, save the soaking water, starch, and bran. It can be used to thicken soups, sauces, stews, puddings, and so on, as well as for pancakes, waffles, and sourdough starter.) Add cold water to the pot and start to knead all the bran out of the gluten.

If this water also becomes overly branny, add fresh water. (Save this bran water as well, if desired.) Start to take small pieces of the gluten, one at a time, and wash the bran out of them. They can be rinsed under the tap. (Some remaining flecks of bran here and there is all right. It need not be prefectly bran-free.)

When finished, separate the gluten into several pieces and drop them into a pot of boiling water until they rise to the surface. (Or, deep-fry them until they puff up and turn golden brown. Try it this way when no longer healing; it is delicous.)

Cook the seitan further if desired. Put a piece of kombu, seitan, ⅓ to ½ cup tamari soy sauce, and 6 cups of spring water into a pot, bring it to a boil, turn flame to low, cover, and simmer for about a half hour. Eat as is or add to other dishes, including soups, salads, vegetables, stews, grains, and the like.

Seitan Stew

> 5 onions, quartered
> 1 rutabaga, cut into $1\frac{1}{2}''$ pieces
> 2 carrots, cut into $1\frac{1}{2}''$ pieces
> 7–10 Brussels sprouts
> Cooked seitan, with tamari broth from recipe
> Finely chopped parsley
> *Optional:* 1–2 cups seitan starch water

In a large pot, layer onions, carrots, rutabaga, seitan pieces, and Brussels sprouts on top. Add enough of the seitan cooking broth to cover seitan. (If the broth is salty, use half water and half broth.) Bring to a boil and simmer, covered, for 20 to 30 minutes, or until the vegetables are tender. Slowly pour seitan starch water into the pot, while stirring constantly. When the stew thickens, simmer for 5 minutes more on low heat. Serve garnished with chopped parsley. Grated ginger, ginger juice, and/or chopped scallions can also be used for a garnish.

This stew is ideal for those with a more yin condition. Serves 6 to 8.

Cabbage, Carrots and Seitan
(This quicker dish is helpful as a replacement for animal food for those with a more yang condition.)

> 2 cups cabbage, cut into 1″ pieces
> 1 cup carrots, sliced on a thin diagonal
> Several seitan pieces
> Water
> *Optional:* ½–1 tsp. tamari soy sauce

Place seitan, carrots, and cabbage in a pot. Add enough water to come to ¼ the height of the vegetables. Add tamari soy sauce, if using. Cover, bring to a boil, and simmer for 5 to 10 minutes, or until the vegetables are tender. Serves 6.

Variations: Other vegetables like snow peas and yellow squash can also be used. Chopped scallions and/or grated ginger can be added after cooking.

Seitan Roast with Mushroom Gravy

1 batch seitan, completely uncooked
2–3 cups starch water (from first rinse)
1 strip kombu, 4″–6″
¼ cup sliced ginger root
5 shiitake mushrooms
Tamari soy sauce
½ cup chopped scallion or parsley

In a large pot, bring about ½ gallon of water to a boil. Soak shiitake and kombu until soft. Slice shiitake, removing the tough stem. Slice kombu. Add shiitake, kombu, and ginger root to water. Season with tamari soy sauce.

Shape uncooked seitan into a round loaf. Place the loaf in the broth and simmer for 1 hour, or until the seitan is cooked all the way through. Remove seitan, slice, and place in a serving dish. Remove ginger slices from broth.

Slowly add starch water to the broth, while stirring constantly. When the broth comes back to a boil, turn heat to low and simmer 5 minutes more. Pour this hot gravy over the seitan roast and serve garnished with chopped parsley or scallion. (Seitan cooked this way can also be used for sandwiches.) Served 5 to 6.

3.   Fu is also a by-product of wheat gluten. It looks like a cracker and is packaged and available in natural food stores. Fu comes in flat sheets or thick rounds which are available in small or large sizes.

Chinese Cabbage and Fu

2 cups Chinese cabbage, cut into 1″ slices
3–4 sheets flat fu, soaked, and cut into ¼″ slices
2 sheets toasted nori, sliced into ½″ strips
1 pinch sea salt
Water

In a small pot, place fu, Chinese cabbage, salt, and about 1½ inches of water. Cover, bring to a boil, and simmer until cabbage is tender (about 10 minutes). Uncover and boil away excess liquid. Mix in nori strips and serve. Serves 3 to 4.

Fu and Broccoli in Broth

1 strip kombu, 6″–8″, soaked
4 5 cups water
1 cup fu, soaked and sliced
1 cup broccoli floweretts and stems
Tamari soy sauce

Put the kombu and water in a pot and bring to a boil. Cover and lower the heat to medium-low. Simmer for about 10 minutes. Remove the kombu, drain, and set aside for future use. Add the fu to the water and simmer for 5 minutes. Add the broccoli and simmer until done. The broccoli should be bright green. When the broccoli is just about done, season with a little tamari soy sauce, and simmer for 2 to 3 minutes longer. Transfer to individual serving bowls and serve while hot.

4. Sourdough bread. When healing, it is best to abstain from baked flour products, as mentioned before, but if you do crave some, natural, unyeasted sourdough bread is best.

    Yeast is not recommended as it can cause indigestion, and can weaken the intestines.

    Hard spring or winter wheat flours make the best bread as they contain much gluten which helps the bread rise. Any other flour can be added in smaller proportions for a variation in taste, as can any cooked grains. (Cooked grains that have already gone sour can replace the sourdough starter.)

    Before making a sourdough bread, you first need to make a starter.

Sourdough Starter

1 cup whole wheat flour
1–1½ cups well or spring water

Put flour and water into a bowl and mix them into a thick batter or porridge-like consistency, adding more flour or water as needed. Cover with a damp towel, and let it sit for 2 to 4 days at room temperature. When it bubbles and becomes sour, it is ready to use.

Sourdough Bread (2 Loaves)

5 cups whole wheat flour
1 cup sourdough starter (or sour seitan water)
2 cups water

1 tsp. sea salt

Mix the starter, water, and 2½ cups of the flour. Let the mixture sit uncovered in a warm place for an hour or so until it rises.

(At this point, half of this batter can be saved for an ongoing starter which can be used continually by adding to and recycling it every week; the longer it has been around the better the bread. If not baking one week, mix in a few spoonfuls of flour and water just to keep the starter going and to prevent it from spoiling. This should be stored in the refrigerator.)

Add the salt and remaining flour, form into a dough, and on a floured board, start kneading the bread, about 350 to 400 times. The more it is kneaded the better it will rise, as the bread gets more and more elastic, glutenous, and smooth. This is the secret to non-yeasted breads.

Place dough into a lightly oiled bowl, cover with a damp towel, and let it sit overnight at room temperature.

The next morning, punch the dough down, knead it for a few minutes, and divide it in half. Place the halves into two oiled bread pans, and with a knife, make a lengthwise slit down the center of the tops. The slit helps to give the bread some room to grow and lets steam escape. Place the pans in a very warm place and let them sit for another 2 to 3 hours or until the bread rises and the slits begin to open.

Make the slits deeper and take an oiled rubber spatula and pull the bread away from the sides of the pans. Bake at 350° to 375° F. for about an hour, or until the bread forms a beautiful brown crust.

Insert a chopstick or fork into the bread and pull it out again. If no flour sticks to it, the bread is done. Also, when tapping the bottom, a hollow sound will be heard if the bread is finished. Remove from the pans and let the loaves cool on a bread rack for several hours. Eating the bread while it is still hot may cause an upset stomach. Keep loaves in a cool, dark place, wrapped in a clean cotton cloth or towel.

Slice with a bread knife. If the bread becomes hard, simply steam the number of slices desired for a few minutes. They will become moist and appear freshly baked.

Rice Kayu Bread

2 cups whole wheat flour

¼ tsp. sea salt
2 cups soured soft rice (Leave soft rice—rice cereal—at room
   temperature for 2 to 4 days and it will naturally sour.)

Mix flour and salt together. Add soft rice and form the dough
into a ball. Knead about 350 to 400 times. Dough should be
smooth and elastic.

Lightly oil a bread pan (you can also dust the oiled pan with
flour), shape the dough into a loaf and place it in the pan.
Cut a slit down the center of the loaf. Cover with a damp
towel and let sit for 8 hours to overnight at room temperature.
(If the towel dries out, you can wet it again.)

Bake in a preheated 250°F oven for 30 minutes. Turn heat
to 350°F and continue to cook for another hour. Test bread
to see if it is done before removing from pan. (*See Sourdough
Bread* recipe, above.) Cool on a wire rack before slicinng.

Sourdough Pancakes

2 cups whole wheat flour
1 cup sourdough starter or slightly sour amazake
¼ tsp. sea salt
Water
Small amount sesame or corn oil

Mix together flour and salt. Add starter or amazake and
enough water to make desired pancake consistency. Stir
thoroughly (about 5 minutes worth). Cover with a damp towel
and let sit overnight in a warm place.

In the morning, heat a skillet on medium heat. Coat the
bottom of the pan with oil, and spoon in pancake batter.
Cook until bubbles rise, break, and do not fill themselves back
up. Flip and cook the other side until it is lightly browned.

Keep the pancakes warm until ready to serve. Eat with fruit
and kuzu sauce, barley-malt kuzu sauce, onion butter or apple
butter. (See *Sauces and Dressings* for more syrup ideas and
recipes.)

Variations: Buckwheat pancakes can be made by using 1 cup
   buckwheat flour and 1 cup whole wheat flour. Corn pancakes or oat pancakes can be made by adding corn meal or
   oatmeal to the batter. This recipe can also be used for making
   waffles as well. By using less liquid, you could also make
   muffins.

8. Soups ━━━━━━━━━━━━━━━━━━━━━━━━━━

Soup at the beginning of a meal prepares the digestive system for all the following dishes. Just about anything can be put into a soup. Practically all types of grains, beans and their products, vegetables, sea vegetables, and occasionally, fish, can be used.

Soups can be adapted seasonally (and be either warming or cooling), and can add contrast to the rest of the meal. There are some general guidelines on deciding what kind of soup to use.

In the winter, make more hearty stews and thick soups with more root vegetables, grains, or beans, and use more salt. In the summer, make lighter soups with less ingredients and more liquid, more greens, tofu, and so on. Also make greater use of clear or light tamari-broth soups in hot weather.

For all stress-related disorders, miso soup with a variety of vegetables and sea vegetables, particularly daikon and green leafy vegetables, should be eaten on a daily basis.

Sweet vegetables such as carrots, onions, squash, parsnips, and cabbage can be used individually or together to make delicious sweet-tasting soups.

Care should be taken to balance soup with the rest of the meal. Some examples are:

1. Make a bean soup for a light meal lacking in more protein-rich dishes such as beans, tempeh, or natto.

2. Make a sweet-vegetable soup (squash, carrots, parsnips, etc.) if the meal is lacking this sweet taste.

3. Make a root-vegetable soup if the meal is mostly greens and vice versa.

4. Make a grain soup to balance a more light meal.

5. Use finely chopped vegetables if the meal contains all big chunks and vice versa.

6. Use a color in the soup which is not represented in the meal.

7. If not making miso soup, miso can be added somewhere else in the meal.

Use a ladle to serve soups. This can be kept on a plate on the counter next to the soup pot or in a bowl during the course of the meal, ready to be used whenever needed.

Especially during the first few months, it is recommended that every day one meal should contain miso soup (unless soft miso rice is eaten that day). Also, every day, at least one soup should contain sea vegetables. Garnishes are important (parsley or scallions) to balance soups as well as for decoration.

1. *Miso soup:* Miso is an indispensible part of the macrobiotic diet. It gives vitality, strengthens the digestive system and blood quality, and improves assimilation of carbohydrates. When healing, eat a small amount every day, particularly in miso soup.

Miso is salty so care must be taken to avoid consuming too much of it at one time. To use, add a flat teaspoonful per cup of liquid, dissolving the miso in a small amount of liquid before adding it to the soup.

Miso should be added at the end of cooking, after all the ingredients have softened, and generally should not be boiled as otherwise many valuable healing enzymes are destroyed. However, it is important that the soup be simmered for a few minutes after the miso is added to help the body assimilate it. If this is not done, tightness can arise.

The recipes below are primarily for mugi (barley) miso, but Hatcho (all soybean) miso may be used on occasion, especially in the winter.

Basic Miso Soup

> **Wakame or kombu, soaked and sliced**
> **½ cup onions, cut in crescents**
> **½ cup carrots, sliced in half-moons**
> **4 cups spring water**
> **4 level tsps. miso**
> **Scallion or parsley garnish**

Soak wakame or kombu for 10 minutes and slice. Boil the slices in water, cutting vegetables in the meantime. Add the vegetables to the boiling water and cook until they are soft, about 10 minutes. Dilute and purée the miso with some of the soup water, turn down the flame, and when the soup has stopped bubbling, gently add and stir the miso purée into the soup. Simmer for 3 to 4 minutes and serve with a garnish. It is important that the soup be light and energetic by keeping vegetables fresh and crispy, being careful not to overcook them.

Wakame and Daikon Miso Soup

¼ cup wakame, washed, soaked, and sliced
½ cup daikon, cut in half-moons
4 cups spring water
4 level tsps. miso
2 scallions, sliced

Follow the recipe for *Basic Miso Soup.* Serves 6.

Other miso soup variations:

1) **Onion and Daikon Miso Soup:** 2 onions, ½ cup daikon, and about 4 inches of wakame.
2) **Mustard Green Miso Soup:** 1 onion, 2 to 4 mustard-green leaves, and about 4 inches of wakame or kombu.
3) **Miso Soup with Root Vegetables:** 1 carrot, 1 onion, ¼ rutabaga, 1 stalk celery, and about 3 inches of wakame or kombu.
4) **Miso Soup with Squash and Onions:** 2 onions, 1 cup winter squash, and about 3 inches of wakame or kombu.
5) **Miso Soup with Roots and Greens:** Use either carrots and carrot tops, daikon and daikon leaves, radish and radish tops, or turnip and turnip greens, with wakame or kombu. Onions could also be added, but are optional.
6) **Miso Soup with Shiitake and Greens:** 1 to 3 shiitake mushrooms, 3 to 5 leaves of green leafy vegetable, and 5 inches of wakame or kombu.
7) **Miso Soup with Tofu:** ½ cake tofu, choice of vegetables, wakame or kombu.
8) **Tempeh Miso Soup:** ½ package of tempeh, 2 onions, and 4 inches of wakame.
9) **Miso Soup with Fu:** 3 sheets flat fu and 1 leek in a kombu stock.
10) **Dulse Miso Soup:** Use dulse in place of wakame or kombu. Try dulse with cabbage and carrots.

Creamy Squash Miso Soup

1 small butternut or buttercup squash, or Hokkaido pumpkin
1 quart water
Pinch of sea salt
2½–4 tsp. miso

Cut squash into 1-inch pieces. Place in a heavy pot with about 1 inch of water and a pinch of sea salt. Cover, bring to a boil, reduce heat to low, and cook until tender (about 15 to 20 minutes). Puree squash with cooking juice in a suribachi or a food mill.

In a pot, mix remaining water with squash puree. Bring to a boil, reduce heat to low and simmer for 5 minutes. Puree miso in a small amount of soup broth. Add to soup, turn heat to very low, and let set for a minute or two before serving. Garnish with chopped parsley or scallion.

Onion Soup

5 medium-sized onions
3–5 tsp. miso
1 quart water
Scallions or parsley for garnish
Optional: **A few drops sesame oil**

Heat a heavy pot and add sesame oil or a very small amount of water. Slice the onions very thin and add to the pot. Cook on a medium heat, stirring occasionally to prevent scorching. When onions are golden brown, add water. Bring to a boil and simmer for 20 minutes. Puree miso and add to soup. Turn heat to low and let set for a minute or so. Serve garnished. Croutons can also be used to garnish this soup.

2. *Clear broth or tamari soy sauce soup:* Light soups are very appealing in the hot summer months or when the rest of the meal is more heavy. A stronger tamari broth is very good as a standard supper soup for noodles, but care should be taken that the soup does not have a markedly salty taste.

For a clear soup, make a stock and add the vegetables and some form of salt. The following guidelines apply to the making of soup stock:

A. To retain the clear color of the stock, use a pinch of sea salt per cup of liquid.

B. A darker soup can be made by using 2 to 3 tablespoons of tamari soy sauce for every four cups of liquid.

C. For occasional use, 1 flat tablespoon of umeboshi paste or 2 umeboshi plums for 4 cups of liquid will give an attractive pink coloring to a soup.

Squash Soup

1 medium-sized buttercup or butternut squash

4 to 5 cups spring water
¼ to ½ tsp. sea salt
Toasted nori, cut into 1″-squares for garnish
Chopped parsley or sliced scallions for garnish

Wash the squash and remove the skin and seeds. Cut the squash into large chunks to obtain 4 to 5 cups. Put the squash in a pot and add the water and a pinch of sea salt. Bring to a boil. Cover, lower the heat, and simmer until the squash is soft, about 40 minutes to an hour. Pour the squash and cooking water into a hand food mill and puree. Return the puréed squash to the pot, season with the remaining sea salt, and simmer for several minutes. Pour the soup into individual serving bowls and garnish with a few squares of toasted nori and chopped parsley or scallions.

Tofu, Watercress, Tamari-Broth Soup

1 cube fresh tofu, cut into smaller cubes
1 bunch watercress, washed
½ carrot, cut into very thin matchsticks
1 onion, cut into very thin half-moons
4 cups soup stock
2–3 Tbsps. tamari soy sauce

Bring the soup stock to a boil, drop in the watercress for 2 seconds and then remove, setting it aside to drain for the time being. Add the carrots and onions until they are soft. Then add the tamari and tofu (until it rises to the top) and simmer over a low flame for 3 to 5 minutes. Dish the soup out into individual bowls and garnish with the boiled watercress (which you may chop into more bite-size slices if you desire). Serves 4.

Cabbage Umeboshi Soup

¼ green cabbage
½ leek, sliced into thin pieces
½ carrot, cut into thin matchsticks
1 qt. kombu stock
2–3 umeboshi plums

Bring stock to a boil. Add cabbage, carrot, and leek. Simmer 3 to 5 minutes or until vegetables are cooked through, but still crunchy. Remove pits from plums and grind remaining plum with a little soup broth in a suribachi. Add to soup and cook for 2 to 3 minutes more. Remove from heat and cool to room temperature or chill slightly. Serve garnished with a parsley sprig or a celery leaf. Serves 4.

3. *Grain and bean soups:* Any combination of fresh or leftover grains and beans can be made into a delicious soup. Fresh beans and grains will of course require a longer cooking time than soups made with leftovers.
   A. Boiling. To boil, layer the vegetables in a pot. Place the more yin vegetables on the bottom and the more yang ones on top (except for greens which are added later and placed on top). Then add the grains or beans, and enough water just to barely cover everything. Bring to a slow boil, adding more water as the grains or beans expand. You can place a heat deflector underneath to help prevent burning. This is the same method used in boiling beans (see *Beans and Bean Products* chapter), except that instead of boiling away the excess liquid in the end, we add more to make it soupy. The salt and/or miso or tamari are added after the grain or bean has softened (simmer another 3 to 10 minutes after the seasoning is added). More water can be added if the consistency is too thick.

   Soaking the grain or bean beforehand shortens the cooking time. If using previously cooked grains or beans, first boil the vegetables until they are soft, and then add the grains or beans. As an option, sauté the vegetables and/or roast the grains or beans beforehand. An optional piece of kombu may be added in the bottom of the pot.

Millet and Squash Soup

Follow the directions for *Millet and Squash* in the *Grains and Grain Products* chapter, except use more water. Other sweet vegetables can also be used. Rice may be used instead of millet.

Split Pea Soup

   1 cup green split peas
   2 onions, diced
   2 carrots, diced
   1 stalk celery, diced
   1 strip kombu, 4", washed and soaked
   2 pinches sea salt
   Miso or tamari soy sauce to taste
   Chopped parsley or scallion for garnish

Cut the kombu and place it on the bottom of the pot. Continue, following directions for *Boiled Grain and Bean Soups*. Add salt after the beans are soft. Add tamari soy sauce towards the end of cooking, or miso at the end of cooking. Garnish with chopped scallion or parsley.

Pressure-cooking: Pressure-cooking grain and bean soups is quicker, though the cooking style is a little more yang. First, pressure-cook grains or beans until soft. Remove the lid and add salt and vegetables. (For grain soups, salt can be added at the beginning. For both soups, kombu or wakame can be added at the beginning.)

Simmer until vegetables are almost tender, adding water as necessary to keep the ingredients covered. Add tamari soy sauce and enough water to make desired soup consistency and continue to cook for 15 to 20 minutes more. If you are using miso, add enough water to make a soup consistency about 20 minutes before the end of cooking, adding miso when soup is done.

Barley Shiitake Soup

$\frac{1}{2}$ **cup barley, soaked 6–8 hours or overnight**
3 shiitake mushrooms, soaked until soft
2 pinches sea salt
5–6 cups water
Tamari soy sauce to taste
$\frac{1}{2}$ **bunch watercress, blanched and cut into 1″ pieces for garnish**

Pressure-cook all ingredients for 40 to 45 minutes. Let the pressure come down completely, uncover, and bring to a boil again. Add tamari soy sauce, turn flame to low, place a flame deflector underneath, and simmer for another 15 minutes. Serve, garnishing each bowl with watercress. Serves 5.

Rice Stew

1 cup short- or medium-grain brown rice
1 pinch sea salt
4 plus 2 cups water
1 onion, cubed
1 carrot, cubed
1 burdock, cubed
1 stem celery, cubed
Miso to taste
Chopped scallions for garnish

Pressure-cook rice with salt and 4 cups of water for 45 minutes. Layer in a heavy pot: kombu, onions, burdock, carrots, and then celery. Pour soft rice over vegetables and add enough water to cover. Slowly bring to a boil and place a flame deflector underneath. Simmer on low heat until all the vegetables are tender, adding more water as necessary. Season with miso, let cook (not boil) for 2 minutes more. Serve, garnishing each bowlful with a generous portion of grated ginger and chopped scallions.

Azuki Bean Soup

1 strip kombu, 4″
1 tsp. fresh grated ginger
1 cup azuki beans
1 cup diced onions
1 cup diced carrots
5–6 cups water
2–4 pinches sea salt
1 strip kombu, 4″–5″
Several parsley sprigs for garnish

Layer the kombu, onions, carrots, and then azuki beans in a pressure cooker. Add water, bring to pressure, and cook for 45 minutes. Let the pressure come down and add sea salt. Simmer for 20 minutes more and serve, garnishing each bowl with parsley. (Tamari soy sauce or miso can also be added.)

4. *Soup Stocks:* These soup stocks can be used for any of the above types of soups. They are particularly good for the clear, miso, and vegetable soups.

Kombu Soup Stock

1 strip kombu, 3″–6″
5–6 cups spring water

Wipe dust from kombu with a clean, damp cloth. Leave the white powder on. Bring the kombu and water to a boil, simmer about 3 minutes, and remove the kombu. It can be reused for another stock (boil it longer the next time to get more out of it), added to another dish, or sliced and used in this one. Other variations:

  a) **4 shiitake mushrooms, simmer 5–6 minutes**
  b) **2 Tbsps. bonito fish flakes, simmer 3–4 minutes**

c) Any combination of kombu, shiitake, and bonito
d) Odds and ends of vegetables such as onion skins, cabbage cores, roots, tops, and so on. Wash well, boil 5 minutes, and discard or use for compost.
e) Other sea vegetables such as wakame and dulse
f) Dry-roast grains such as rice, sweet rice, millet, buckwheat, or barley until a nutty fragrance is emitted, and use for stock. Simmer 4–5 minutes.
g) *Chirimen iriko* (small, whole dried fish available in natural and Oriental food stores). Boil 2 Tbsps. 3–4 minutes.
h) Leftover liquid from boiling vegetables
i) Water left over from cooking beans
j) Diluted water left over from cooking seitan

9. Beans and Bean Products ━━━━━

Beans are high in protein and are a delicious addition to your diet. It is important not to overeat beans, to chew them very well, and to cook them thoroughly, otherwise they can cause gas, intestinal problems, and a sluggish condition. Beans should always be a side dish, not compromising more than 15 percent of the meal. As they make a heavier dish, beans are more appropriate for supper, somewhat less often for lunch, and generally not for breakfast.

Azuki beans, chick-peas, lentils, and black soybeans are the most yang beans and the best ones to use on a regular basis. Use these beans, and/or bean products such as tofu and tempeh, about three to six times a week (but in small quantities) when healing. Other beans such as pintos, kidneys, black beans, and red lentils can be eaten occasionally, about once a week or less during the healing process, or may be avoided altogether for several months. Soybeans (which are full of protein) need particular attention so that they are cooked thoroughly. They are delicious in combination with vegetables. They can also be eaten in the form of tofu, tempeh, natto, miso, and tamari soy sauce.

When washing beans, first spread them out a little at a time and remove stones or anything else that may be mixed in. Then place the beans in a bowl, cover them with water, and stir. Rinse off any dust that may rise to the surface. Repeat this about 3 times or until the water becomes clear. When lifting beans out of the water into a strainer or colander to drain, leave out any heavy dust or residue that remains in the bottom of the bowl.

Except for red and green lentils, beans may be soaked for a few hours or overnight prior to cooking. This softens them and helps to cook them quicker. Azuki beans need only a few hours of soaking, and from time to time may be cooked without soaking, particularly when trying to strengthen an overly yin condition. Soaking is preferred for pinto and kidney beans for more digestibility. Chick-peas and soybeans should always be soaked, as they are particularly tough. Use the soaking water as part of the cooking liquid.

Salt is to be added towards the end of the cooking process after the beans have already softened, otherwise they will remain hard. Placing a piece of kombu on the bottom of the pot also helps to soften them, and adds additional minerals and flavor.

There are three main ways to cook beans.

1. *Boiling:* This is the method I prefer the most as it cooks the beans gently, slowly, and thoroughly. Beans turn out really delicious and much sweeter when boiled.

Soak the beans for a few hours or overnight (not necessary for lentils and split peas). Place an optional piece of kombu on the bottom of a pot, then your choice of optional vegetables and finally the beans on top. Add enough water to just cover the beans. Place a drop top inside the pot to sit directly on the beans. This top should be loose fitting to let steam escape on the sides but large enough to cover the inside of the pot as much as possible.

As the beans expand, slowly and gently pour more *cold* water down the sides of the pot from time to time, always enough to just cover them. The sudden cold water helps the beans to soften more quickly. Bring this to a boil over a medium flame.

Then, turn the flame to medium-low and let it simmer for 45 minutes to an hour or so, continuing to add cold water once in a while. Watch closely to see when more water is needed to prevent burning. Do not stir or mix at all, letting the cooking go on undisturbed. This makes for a tastier dish.

When the beans are 70 percent done, add salt and/or miso or tamari soy sauce, remove the drop top, and simmer for another 10 to 20 minutes, or until the beans are completely soft, boiling away any excess liquid.

Azuki Beans, Squash, and Kombu
(Gives vitality, strengthens spleen, pancreas, stomach, and digestion.)

1 cup azuki beans
1 piece kombu, 3″ long
2 cups buttercup or acorn squash or Hokkaido pumpkin
Spring water
2 pinches sea salt

Wash and soak the azuki beans with the kombu for 4 to 5 hours. Remove the kombu and chop it into small squares. Place the kombu in the bottom of a pot and add the squash which has been cut into cubes. Cover the squash with the beans, and add water to just cover the squash layer.

Do not cover the beans at the beginning. Place the bean mixture over low heat and bring to a boil slowly. Cover after about 10 to 15 minutes. Cook until the beans are 70 to 80 percent done, about 1 hour or more.

The water will evaporate as the beans expand, so add cold water occasionally to keep the water level constant. Add sea salt and cook until the beans are done and most of the liquid has evaporated, approximately 15 to 30 minutes more. Transfer to a serving bowl and serve.

Basic Black Soybeans

2 cups black soybeans
6 cups cold spring water
$\frac{1}{4}$ tsp. sea salt
$1\frac{1}{4}$–$1\frac{1}{2}$ Tbsps. tamari soy sauce

Wash the beans with cold water very quickly and put them in a bowl. Cover with about 6 cups of water. Add sea salt and let the beans soak for several hours or overnight.

Put the beans in a pot with the salted soaking water and bring to a boil. Reduce the heat to medium-low and simmer until the beans are about 90 percent done. During the simmering, add water when necessary as the liquid evaporates. As the beans cook, skim off and discard any skins that float to the surface, as well as any gray foam that surfaces.

When the beans are about 90 percent done, add the tamari

soy sauce. Shake the pot gently up and down to evenly coat the beans with the juice and tamari. Do not mix with a spoon. Shaking gives the skins a very shiny black appearance. Cook until almost all the remaining liquid has evaporated.

Total cooking time for this dish is about $2\frac{1}{2}$ to 3 hours.

Lentils

1 cup dried lentils
2–$2\frac{1}{2}$ cups spring water
1 cup diced onion
$\frac{1}{2}$ cup diced celery
1 cup diced carrots
$\frac{1}{4}$ cup diced burdock
$\frac{1}{4}$ tsp. sea salt, or $1\frac{1}{2}$ tsps. tamari soy sauce
Parsley for garnish

Wash the lentils. Make layers of the onions, celery, carrots, and burdock in a pot. Put the lentils on top and add the water. Bring to a boil, reduce the heat to medium-low, and cover. Simmer for 40 to 45 minutes. Season and simmer for another 10 to 15 minutes. Transfer to a serving bowl and garnish with parsley and serve.

2. *Pressure-cooking:* This is the best method for chick-peas as they are extremely hard and tough. Azuki, pinto, and kidney beans can also be pressure-cooked.

Red and green lentils, split peas, and black and white soybeans may clog the pressure gauge of the pressure cooker and cause a possible explosion, so it is best to boil them. In the case of the lentils and split peas, it does not matter much as they soften very quickly anyway. With soybeans, there are three things you can do to make them safer for pressure-cooking.

A. Boil the (presoaked) soybeans and skim off all the foam that rises to the top. When no more foam appears (maybe in a half hour), place them in a pressure cooker and cook till done.

B. Dry-roast the soybeans before pressure-cooking them. Combining black soybeans with rice or another grain, in addition to the roasting, helps even further.

C. Soak black soybeans for several hours or overnight with ⅛ teaspoon of sea salt for every cup of beans. This helps to prevent the skins from coming off and clogging the gauge.

Pinto Beans with Carrots and Onions

1 cup pinto beans
1 strip kombu, 4″–8″
1½ cups carrots, cut into ½″ pieces
1 cup onions, cut into ½″ pieces
1½ tsp. barley miso

Wash and soak beans for 6 to 8 hours. Clean kombu by wiping off any dust with a clean cloth. Place kombu on the bottom of a pressure cooker and proceed as in *Pressure Cooking Method.* Add miso about ½ hour before the end of cooking.

Chick-Peas and Roasted Rice

1 cup brown rice
1 2″-strip kombu
1 cup chick-peas, soaked 8 hours
5 cups spring water
2 pinches sea salt

Dry-roast the rice in a frying pan. Combine the beans and rice in a pot with the kombu underneath. Add the water and bring the beans and rice to a boil. Lower the heat, cover the pot, and simmer until the beans are 70 to 80 percent done. Uncover, season with sea salt, cover the pot, and cook until the beans are soft. When done, remove the cover, turn up the heat and boil off any excess water. Transfer the mixture to a serving bowl and serve.

Colorful Soybean Casserole

(This is a delicious dish which is helpful for overall stamina and sexual vitality.)

2 cups yellow soybeans
Water
1 strip kombu, 6″
1 shiitake mushroom
5 large pieces dried lotus root
6 pieces dried tofu
1 stalk celery, sliced
$\frac{1}{2}$ cup shredded, dried daikon
1 carrot, sliced
1 burdock, sliced
1 pinch sea salt
$1\frac{1}{2}$ Tbsps. tamari soy sauce
1 tsp. kuzu
Fresh grated ginger
Optional: 1–2 Tbsps. mirin

Soak the soybeans overnight in 5 cups of cold water. Next day, put the beans and soaking water in a pressure cooker. Boil the beans uncovered for 15 to 20 minutes. Skim off any foam or hulls. Secure lid, bring to pressure and cook on a low heat for about 20 minutes.

Soak kombu, shiitake, lotus root, and dried tofu for 10 minutes. When the pressure has come down, add to soybeans and pressure-cook 10 to 15 minutes more. Reduce pressure, remove vegetables, kombu, and tofu. Slice. In a heavy pot, layer the kombu, celery, shiitake, dried daikon, tofu, carrot, burdock, and lotus root. Add soybeans on top. Add cooking water and a pinch of sea salt. Cover, and cook for $\frac{1}{2}$ hour or until the celery and carrots are tender. Season with tamari soy sauce.

Dissolve kuzu in a small amount of cold water and add to beans. Cook 5 to 10 minutes more. Just before serving, add fresh grated ginger. Mirin can also be added right at the end of cooking for a sweeter taste.

3. _Baking:_ Baking is a delicious way to cook beans in the winter as it is very hearty.

This method takes the longest time to prepare but the results are well worth the wait. Pintos, kidneys, and soybeans yield well to baking.

To prepare, first place the presoaked beans in a pot on top of the stove, adding 4 to 5 cups of water for every cup of beans. Bring this to a boil, and boil for 15 to 20 minutes to loosen the bean skins.

Then, pour the beans and liquid into a baking pot. (You can place an optional piece of kombu underneath.) Cover, place in the oven, and bake at 350°F., adding more water from time to time as needed. They may be done in about 3 to 4 hours, depending on the type of beans used.

You may add some vegetables halfway through. The salt and/or tamari or miso should be added after the beans have become soft and creamy. After adding the salt, you can take the cover off and let the beans brown a bit. Then, remove from the stove and serve.

Azuki Beans and Chestnuts

2 cups soaked azuki beans
1 cup dried chestnuts, soaked
2 pinches sea salt
8 cups water
1 strip kombu, 3"–6"

Bake, following the above directions.

Variations: (Pressure-cooking or boiling is preferable)

1. Azuki beans with carrots and onions
2. Azuki beans with chestnuts
3. Azuki beans with parsnips
4. Azuki beans with lotus seeds
5. Azuki beans with raisins or rice syrup (for a more yang condition)
6. Chick-peas, plain
7. Chick-peas with carrots and onions
8. Lentils, plain
9. Lentils with winter squash
10. Black soybeans with onions, carrots, and celery
11. Kidney beans with onions
12. Navy beans with onions, carrots, burdock, and celery
13. Lima beans with seitan and onions
14. Any bean recipe cooked with extra water to make soup. (Miso or tamari soy sauce can be added toward the

end of cooking.) Do not use sweetened azuki beans for soup.
15. There are many other bean and vegetable combinations you can make.

Three Bean Salad
(Usually, different beans are not cooked together as the combination may be difficult to digest—it could preduce gas and/or intestinal cramping. This salad, however, is different because two of the beans are vegetables, very different from dried beans.)

1 cup chick-peas cooked with 3″ strip kombu
1 cup diced green string beans, par-boiled
1 cup diced yellow wax beans, par-boiled
1 Tbsp. umeboshi vinegar
½ cup minced parsley

Mix all ingredients together and let marinate for 1 to 2 hours before serving.

Hummus

1 cup chick-peas cooked with 3″ strip kombu
Any leftover water from cooking chick-peas
1 cup finely chopped scallions
½ cup minced parsley
¼–½ cup chopped sauerkraut

Puree chick-peas in a hand food mill or a suribachi. (Add water as needed to obtain desired consistency.) Mix in scallions, parsley, and sauerkraut. Serve as a dip, or salad style with a summer meal. Hummus also makes a nice spread for rice cakes, bread, or sandwiches.

Bean Products:

While healing, it is best not to overconsume bean products. Have a small amount 2 to 3 times a week, frequently substituting dried for fresh tofu during the healing process.

1. Tofu or soybean curd comes in two forms, fresh and dried. The fresh tofu available in Oriental shops is usually prepared using a modern chemicalized curdling agent and it is best to buy natural tofu curdled with *nigari* (which comes from sea salt). This is available in natural food stores, and now in many supermarkets. Dried

Fig. 8   Tofu

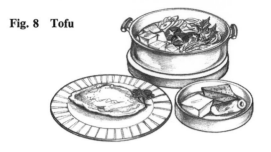

tofu is more strengthening and can be kept indefinitely. Fresh tofu is more yin and should always be cooked.

a)   *Fresh tofu:*   After buying fresh tofu, open the package and store the tofu in the refrigerator submerged in fresh water (throw out the water it came in). Before cooking with it, very quickly rinse the tofu under the tap.

Tofu cooks very quickly and can be boiled, steamed, baked or broiled, sautéed or pan-fried. It is actually done as soon as it is heated up. It can be prepared in many ways.

Pan-fried, Baked or Broiled Tofu

1 cake tofu
Some kind of seasoning (tamari soy sauce, miso, sea salt)
Garnish
***Optional:*   A small amount of sesame oil or water**

Cut tofu into slabs, about ½-inch thick. For sautéing, heat a small amount of sesame oil or water in a skillet. Brown tofu on either side. You can also do this in a dry, cast-iron skillet. Heat the pan first.

For baking or broiling, a small amount of water or sesame oil can be used, but neither is necessary. Brown on both sides.

Tofu cooks quickly, so be careful not to burn it.
Before, after, or during cooking you may spread, dip, or marinate each slice in one of several sauces or dips including: 1) grated ginger and tamari soy sauce, 2) roasted sesame seeds, tamari soy sauce, and chopped scallions, 3) diluted miso and grated ginger, chopped scallions and/or minced onions.

Boiled Tofu with Chinese Cabbage and Carrots

1 cake tofu
3–5 Chinese cabbage leaves cut into 1″ slices
1 carrot cut into very thin slices
2–3 cups water

1 strip kombu, 3″–6″
1 Tbsp. tamari soy sauce
2–3 chopped scallions
1 tsp. grated ginger

Make a kombu stock by boiling, then simmering kombu in water for 3 to 5 minutes. Remove kombu and save for another use. Place carrots, Chinese cabbage, and tofu into separate sections of the pot and boil them for a few minutes until they are done. Make a dip by taking 1 tablespoon of the stock and mixing in the tamari soy sauce, scallions, and ginger. Serves 2 to 3.

Tofu and Seitan Stew

$\frac{1}{2}$ cake tofu, cut in 1″ cubes
1 cup seitan, cut in 1″ cubes
1 strip kombu, 4″
2 carrots, cut in 1″ pieces
1 celery stalk, cut in 1″ pieces
1 burdock root, cut in 1″ pieces
1 onion, sliced in 1″ crescents
A few pinches of sea salt
Tamari soy sauce to taste
Chopped scallion or grated ginger for garnish

Soak kombu until soft and cut it into 1-inch pieces. Place the pieces in a pot, add the burdock, and cover with water. (Use the soaking water from the kombu.) Cover, bring to a boil, and simmer for 10 minutes. Remove burdock. Layer on top of kombu: onions, burdock, carrots, seitan, celery, and then tofu. Cover with water and add salt. Bring to a boil and simmer until all the vegetables are tender and the tofu is cooked. Season with tamari soy sauce a few minutes before the end of cooking. Serve, garnished with ginger or scallion.

Variations: Many other vegetables can be used instead of those listed above. Dried tofu can be substituted for fresh. (Put it at the bottom of the pot.) Kuzu can be added at the end for a thicker stew. More water can be used to make a soup, less to make a vegetable dish.

Scrambled Tofu and Corn

3 Tbsps. dark sesame or corn oil
16 ozs. firm tofu
3 cups fresh sweet corn kernels, removed from the cob

½–1 tsp. sea salt
Sliced scallions for garnish

Heat the oil in a pot. Crumble the tofu and add it to the pot.
Put the sweet corn on top of the tofu. Cover and cook over
low heat for 3 to 4 minutes, or until the tofu becomes hot and
the corn is done. Sprinkle a small amount of sea salt on top
of the corn. Mix and serve hot. Just before serving, add scallions as a garnish, but, to retain their bright green color, do
not cook them.

Variations: The tofu, corn, and scallions may also be sautéed
in 2 to 3 tablespoons of water for those who need to limit their
oil. Other vegetables may be added or substituted, including
cabbage, onions, carrots (cut into matchsticks), and so on. The
colors of the vegetables should be bright, and the texture
slightly crispy.

Pickled Tofu
(An unusual but absolutely delicious dish, very similar in taste
to cheese.)

1 cake firm tofu
Enough miso to coat tofu

Completely cover tofu with a ¼-inch layer of miso. Let this
sit (refrigerate in summer) for 1 to 3 days. The longer the tofu
pickles, the more miso-flavored and salty it will become.
Scrape off miso and save for another use. Thoroughly rinse
tofu before serving. You can also cook tofu before pickling.
Fair Warning: Only make a small amount at a time, it is
very easy to over eat.

b) *Dried tofu:* Dried tofu can be bought at natural or Oriental
food stores. It looks like thin, lightly yellow, rectangular wafers.
To cook, first soak it in water until it softens. Then cut it into
any desired size or leave it whole. This can be combined with
vegetables and treated like one of them. It should be boiled at
least 15 minutes. Dried tofu can also be pressure-cooked and
used in soups and stews.

Dried Tofu, Carrots, and Onions

2 Tbsps. dark sesame oil (optional)
1 cup onions, sliced into half-moons
1 cup carrots, cut into matchsticks
Spring water

1 cup dried tofu, soaked and sliced
2 tsps. tamari soy sauce

Heat the sesame oil in a frying pan and add the onions. (Or water-sauté the onions in a small amount of spring water.) Add the carrots and enough water to cover the bottom of the pan. Add the sliced tofu and sauté for 1 to 2 minutes. Bring to a boil. Add a little tamari soy sauce. Reduce the heat to low and cover.

Simmer for several minutes, or until the carrots and onions are done. Season with a little more tamari soy sauce, mix and sauté until all the liquid has evaporated. Transfer to a serving bowl and serve.

2. *Tempeh:* Tempeh is a fermented soy product used in Indonesia and available in most natural food stores. It is energizing and full of protein. Store it in the refrigerator.

Tempeh can be cooked from a few minutes to 30 minutes or more. The longer it is cooked, the more digestible and smoother-tasting it becomes.

In boiling, steaming, pressure-cooking, baking, and sautéing with vegetables, pan- or deep-fry the tempeh beforehand, to make the dish especially delicious. Tempeh can be deep-fried without any batter or covering. Unlike fresh tofu, add it to dishes in the beginning of the cooking preparation.

Tempeh with Vegetables
(This dish is helpful for those with a more yin condition.)

1 pkg. tempeh
2 carrots
1 small rutabaga (unwaxed)
1 burdock root
2 onions
1 strip kombu, 5″
2–4 pinches sea salt

Wash all vegetables and cut into 1½-inch pieces. Cut tempeh approximately the same size. Wipe kombu with a cloth to clean, and soak for 20 minutes. Slice kombu in 1½-inch pieces and place them on the bottom of a heavy pot. Add onion, tempeh, burdock, carrot, and rutabaga on top. Add about 2 inches of water and sea salt. Cover, bring to a boil, reduce heat to medium-low, and cook for 20 to 30 minutes, or until all vegetables are tender and the tempeh is done. This can be served with chopped scallions for garnish.

Variations: Dried tofu or seitan can be used with or instead of tempeh. Other vegetables can be used: cabbage, leeks, parsnip, Brussels sprouts, cauliflower, broccoli (added toward the end of cooking), and so on. This dish could be pressure-cooked as well. To make this dish more appropriate for those with a more yang condition, use lighter vegetables along with the root vegetables, adding them toward the end of cooking: broccoli, string beans, scallions, shiitake mushrooms can be added at the beginning, celery, leeks, and so on are examples.

Cabbage-Roll Tempeh

5–6 green cabbage or Chinese cabbage leaves, lightly steamed
5–6 pieces tempeh, 2″ by 3″
Spring water
Tamari soy sauce
Small amount sesame oil
5–6 toothpicks
1 strip kombu, 8″, soaked
Kuzu
Sliced scallions for garnish
***Optional:* Grated fresh ginger**

Pan-fry tempeh with or without a small amount of oil until golden on either side. Place in a saucepan and cover with water. Add tamari soy sauce for a mild salt taste and ½ teaspoon grated ginger. Bring to a boil, cover, and reduce heat to low. Simmer for 15 to 20 minutes, remove, and drain.

Wrap each piece of tempeh in a cabbage leaf and fasten with a toothpick. Place kombu in the bottom of a skillet and add cabbage rolls. Add water to half the height of the cabbage rolls. Bring to a boil, cover, and simmer for a short time. (For softer cabbage rolls, cook longer.)

Remove cabbage rolls and arrange on a serving dish. Thicken the remaining cooking water with kuzu which has been dissolved in a small amount of cold water. (Stir constantly to prevent lumping.) Season with a small amount of tamari and a little grated ginger. Pour over cabbage rolls and serve.

Tempeh Sandwich

4 slices sourdough bread
Tempeh
Sauerkraut
1 strip kombu, 4″

Chopped scallions or onion slices
Lettuce
Sprouts
Tamari soy sauce
Optional: 1 tsp. sesame oil

Heat oil or water in a skillet and sauté the tempeh on either side until golden brown. Place kombu in the bottom of a pot, then add tempeh and sauerkraut. Cover with water, bring to a boil, and simmer for 25 minutes. Season with a small amount of tamari soy sauce and continue to cook until the water is gone. Steam, toast, or use bread as is. Make a sandwich with lettuce, sprouts, tempeh, and the sauerkraut the tempeh was cooked with.

Variations: Tempeh can be deep-fried or boiled plain. Other fillings can be used with the tempeh, like cucumber, grated carrot, sautéed onion, tofu dressing, other kinds of pickles instead of sauerkraut, and so on. A very rich sandwich can be made by cooking mochi with the tempeh. Slice mochi into very thin slices. Lay on top of the tempeh for the last 15 to 20 minutes of cooking, letting the mochi melt over the tempeh.

Seitan, tofu, and bean spreads can also be used to make delicious sandwiches.

3. *Natto:* Natto is a stringy, fermented, soybean product. At first, the smell may be unpleasant to some individuals. However, once a taste is acquired for natto, many people cannot get enough of it.

Natto is rich in protein and vitamin B_{12}; it imparts vitality and is easily digested and assimilated. It can be purchased at natural or Oriental food stores. Natto generally comes frozen; thaw it by leaving it in the refrigerator for a day, or at room temperature for a few hours.

To serve, stir in one or more of the following ingredients: 1) grated daikon, 2) grated ginger, 3) chopped scallions, or 4) diced raw onions with the addition of either tamari soy sauce, umeboshi paste, or sauerkraut. Pieces of nori may also be mixed in. These combinations may be eaten on top of rice or other grains as a condiment, or in miso soup.

10. Vegetables ━━━━━━━━━━

As much as possible, get organically grown, chemical-free vegetables. Besides being healthier, they are more delicious. Organic farmers put much care and attention into producing food that benefits both mankind and the planet. Also, avoid dull-colored, limp, yellow-leafed, soft, spotted, or wrinkled items, as they are either too old, spoiled, dried up and/or lacking in vitality.

Choose locally grown produce as often as possible, though in the north during the winter more southern-grown ones will be eaten. Prepackaged items tend to spoil more quickly. Stay away from canned and frozen foods. They have no energy and/or have added salt, sugar, and preservatives, all of which are best avoided. Also, be careful not to buy waxed items.

At home, immediately remove any yellow leaves and spoiled parts of your vegetables before storing them. This helps to preserve the rest for a longer time. When storing vegetables in the refrigerator, keep them in a paper bag; this allows them to absorb extra moisture and thereby retards spoilage. A plastic bag retains water, does not allow your vegetables to breathe, and causes them to grow soggy and spoil more quickly. Keep vegetables separated from fruits for better preservation.

Do not wash vegetables until just before cooking. Any soil left on them helps to keep them fresh longer. When washing vegetables, particularly the leafy greens, it helps to submerge them in a big bowl of water. Gently swish them and then wash each leaf individually. This automatically separates and loosens the sand, soil, and dirt which settles to the bottom of the bowl, as the greens stay afloat. This is much more effective and easier than just trying to rinse them under the tap. Roots can be scrubbed gently with a vegetable brush (*tawashi*) to remove any soil, but make sure to keep the skin on. (Do not peel organic vegetables, as they are not sprayed, or covered with wax. The skins contain many nourishing nutrients.)

To wash leeks, cut them in half lengthwise, and clean out all the dirt trapped between the layers of leaves. The soil usually collects in the section where the colors change from white to green.

Always use cold water when cleaning vegetables as hot water washes out many vitamins and minerals. Wash vegetables quickly. Soaking for any length of time also depletes valuable nutrients.

Within one dish, cut your vegetables uniformly for even cooking. Within a meal, have a variety of different sizes represented in several dishes—smaller for sautéed items, and bigger chunks for stews, for example.

Save the tops and roots of vegetables. They can be cleaned, chopped very finely, and incorporated into vegetable dishes. You can also leave them uncut and use them in a soup stock. Using the whole plant helps to create a balance in your system.

I recommend the square, Japanese vegetable knives (see *Cookware* chapter) for cutting vegetables. They are very handy, flexible, and easy to use. With these knives, we do not cut straight down, or use them like a saw. Starting with the front tip or edge, gently slide the length of the blade across your vegetables in one smooth stroke. *Important: Always Keep Your Fingertips Curled Underneath So That Your Knuckles Show When You Are Cutting.* This helps to protect the fingers from accidental cuts and slips, and allows a better grip on the vegetable as well.

There are several cutting styles to choose from. Here is a partial listing.

1)	Round slices	7)	Matchsticks
2)	Diagonal slices	8)	Shavings
3)	Triangular shapes	9)	Cubing, dicing, and mincing
4)	Rectangles	10)	Wedge slices
5)	Half-moons	11)	Slicing cabbages
6)	Quarters	12)	Slicing big leafy greens

Fig. 9   Vegetable Cutting Styles

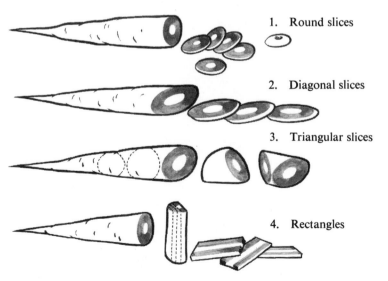

1. Round slices

2. Diagonal slices

3. Triangular slices

4. Rectangles

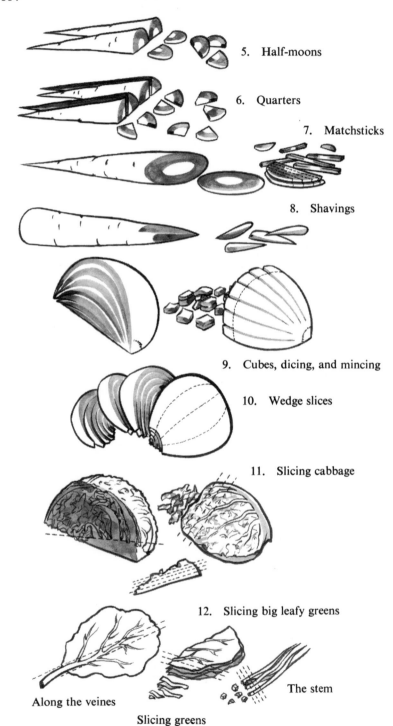

5. Half-moons

6. Quarters

7. Matchsticks

8. Shavings

9. Cubes, dicing, and mincing

10. Wedge slices

11. Slicing cabbage

12. Slicing big leafy greens

Along the veines

The stem

Slicing greens

Include a variety of different kinds of vegetables (roots, greens, ground, and sea vegetables, for example) in a meal as well as an assortment of textures, and colors. Also, use a variety of cooking styles. Here are some of the main methods that we use.

1. *Boiling methods:* There are two main styles of boiling: quick, short-time, and slow, longer-time boiling. Some kind of boiled vegetable can be served at nearly every meal.

   A. Quick boiling (blanching): Blanching is the best way to cook leafy green vegetables. Fill a pot with 1 to 2 inches of water and bring to a boil. Dip in vegetables and take them out quickly. An oil skimmer lifts them easily. Drain the vegetables in a colander. Place a plate underneath to catch excess liquid which can be put back into the pot. Chinese cabbage, broccoli, cauliflower, celery, and others can be used.

   The main point in this style is to cook in as short a time as possible, retaining crispness and bright colors. For example, watercress can be taken out after 15 to 30 seconds. Others take a little longer, in varying degrees, but not much more.

   A pinch of salt in the water helps retain bright colors (but leave it out when cooking bitter vegetables such as watercress and mustard greens, as salt will hold in the bitter flavor).

   Root vegetables can also be cooked in this way but you have to cut them into very thin slices. Boil them for a slightly longer time than you would with greens.

   If you want to boil several different vegetables, do them one by one. Start with the lighter-tasting varieties like the cabbages, and end with more strong-tasting ones like mustard greens, so that the flavor of the latter will not overpower the flavor of the former. Each vegetable's distinct individuality should be maintained.

   You can use the leftover boiling water as a base for a soup. Or you can add some kuzu to it (2 teaspoons for one cup water) to thicken it into a sauce to pour over your vegetables. To do this, first dilute the kuzu in a small amount of cold water. Turn the flame to low under the boiled water and pour the kuzu in. Stir and simmer until the liquid turns clear. Add a little tamari soy sauce or umeboshi paste to taste, and pour this over boiled vegetables.

Boiled Kale

1 small bunch kale

4 cups water
1 pinch sea salt

Bring water and salt to a boil. Thoroughly wash the kale. Boil whole leaves, a few at a time, until they are bright green and just tender. Remove and drain. When cool, cut to desired size.

Boiled Salad

$\frac{1}{2}$ **Chinese cabbage, separated into leaves**
1 bunch watercress
1 onion, cut in thin crescents
1 carrot, cut in matchsticks
1 stalk celery, cut on the diagonal
Spring water
Toasted, ground sesame seeds for garnish

Bring 1 to 2 inches of spring water to a boil with a pinch of sea salt. Boil the vegetables separately in the following order, rinsing each in cold water after they are removed from the pot: Chinese cabbage leaves (1 to 2 minutes); onions (1 minute); carrots (2 minutes); celery (1 minute); watercress (10 seconds).

Slice the cabbage leaves and watercress in thin crosswise slices, mix all vegetables together, adding the toasted sesame seeds and a little rice vinegar, if desired.

B.   Slow, longer-time boiling: Slow boiling is basically for root vegetables such as daikon, carrots, onions, lotus root, burdock, and so on, as well as for squash. This style gives a calming but strong and healing energy.

One or two pieces of kombu are usually placed in the bottom of the pot to help prevent the vegetables from burning, to add extra minerals and flavor, and to help harmonize all the ingredients.

The vegetables are then layered on top of the kombu, with the more yin ones on the bottom and the more yang ones on the top. The yin rising energy meets the yang descending energy and the dish is better integrated.

If the vegetables are fairly dry, put in enough water to just cover them. If they are fresh and more watery, cover them only halfway with water. Add a pinch of salt, cover the pot, bring everything to a boil, turn the flame to low, and simmer for about 20 minutes, or until soft. The time depends on the type, quality, and slice sizes of the vegetables used. Do not mix or stir the vegetables. When the vegetables are soft, add some tamari soy sauce for more flavor, and simmer another 5 minutes. Shiitake mushrooms, dried tofu, tempeh, and seitan may also be added to this dish.

Califlower, Carrots, and Leeks

1 small cauliflower, separate the individual flowers
2 carrots, cut into triangular wedges
2 leeks, cut into triangular wedges (as much as possible)
  Separate the white stem from the green leaves
1 strip kombu, 3″
1 pinch sea salt
Enough water to half cover the vegetables
Optional: **Tamari soy sauce to taste**

Place the kombu in the bottom of the pot. Add the white bottom of the leeks, then the carrots, cauliflower, and the leek greens on top. Add water and salt, cover, and follow the above directions, cooking for 12 to 15 minutes, or until all the vegetables are tender. Serves 4 to 5.

Daikon and Kombu

Daikon radish, cut into 1″ rounds
Kombu

Wash kombu and soak until tender. Slice into 1-inch pieces and place them in the bottom of a pot. Add daikon on top and enough water to come to half the height of the vegetables. Add a pinch of sea salt and cook as described in *Slow, Longer-Time Boiling.*

2. *Nishime style:* Nishime is a medicinal form of cooking using a minimal amount of water. For this, either a heavy pot with a heavy lid or some cookware designed for waterless cooking is needed.

Kombu at the bottom of the pot helps to prevent burning as well as adding extra minerals and taste.

Root vegetables such as carrots, daikon, turnips, burdock, lotus root, onions, and hard winter squash (acorn, buttercup, or Hokkaido), cabbage, and shiitake mushrooms are often used. For reproductive disorders, the use of sweet vegetables should be emphasized. The vegetables are layered on top of the kombu from yin to yang (yin on the bottom). Squash dissolves and loses its shape if cooked for a long time, so it can be added a little later on.

To cook, soak a piece of kombu until it is soft, cut it into

1-inch squares, and place it in the bottom of a pot. Add enough water just to cover the kombu if the vegetables are fresh and watery. If they are more dry, or if using burdock or lotus root, add enough water to cover the vegetables halfway. Put in the vegetables and sprinkle a pinch or two of sea salt or a few drops of tamari soy sauce over them.

Cover, set the flame on high until a steam is produced. Then lower the flame and let the vegetables simmer peacefully for 15 to 20 minutes. If water should evaporate during cooking, add a little more to the bottom of the pot if it is necessary to prevent burning.

When all the vegetables have softened, add a few more drops of tamari soy sauce to taste.

Then, replace the cover, and cook over a low flame for 2 to 5 minutes more. After turning off the flame, remove the cover and let the vegetables sit for about 2 minutes. Serve the juice along with the vegetables as it is very delicious.

Squash, Cabbage, Onion, and Kombu

1 pinch sea salt
Water
$\frac{1}{2}$ buttercup squash, cut into 2"-chunks
$\frac{1}{4}$ cabbage, cut into 2"-squares
2 onions, quartered
1 strip kombu, 5", washed, soaked and cut into 2"-pieces
1 pinch sea salt
Tamari soy sauce to taste
Just enough water to cover the kombu

Follow the directions for *Nishimi Style*. Serves 4 to 6.

Carrots and Parsnips

3 carrots, cut into triangular shapes
3 parsnips, cut into triangular shapes
1 strip kombu, 4"
1 pinch sea salt

Follow the directions for *Nishime Style*. Serves 4 to 6.
Variations:
1. Omit sea salt, just using kombu and optional tamari soy sauce.
2. Omit kombu, just using sea salt and optional tamari soy sauce.
3. Carrot, cabbage, burdock, and kombu

4. Daikon, shiitake mushrooms, and kombu
5. Carrots, lotus root, burdock, and kombu
6. Onions and kombu
7. Parsnips, onions, and kombu
8. Winter squash, onions, and kombu
9. Tempeh, carrot, onion, rutabaga, and Brussels sprouts with kombu
10. Mix in chopped parsley, scallions, or grated ginger at the end of cooking.
11. Add kuzu to remaining cooking water to make a sauce for the vegetables.

Turnips with Greens

Turnips with greens
1 3″-piece kombu, soaked and sliced
Miso or tamari soy sauce to taste
Enough spring water to just cover the kombu

Wash and finely slice the turnips and greens. Put the kombu in a pot with enough water to just cover it. Add the turnips, cover, and cook with a high steam for 10 minutes or longer. Toward the end, add the greens, miso or tamari soy sauce to taste, and simmer for another 2 to 4 minutes.

Other variations:

1) **Daikon and its greens**
2) **Carrots and their greens (slice greens extra fine)**
3) **Radish and its leaves**
4) **Dandelion root and leaves**

3. *Sautéing:* There are two ways to sauté: with oil or using water as a substitute. When limiting the use of oil, use the water-sautéing method as often as desired. For this method, instead of using oil, as discussed below, simply add a few tablespoons of water to a frying pan, bring to a boil, and simmer the vegetables until they are soft.

When using oil, it is best to use only sesame oil (particularly the dark or roasted variety) and to spread it onto the bottom of a heated pan with a brush, rather than to pour it in. Put oil into a cast-iron skillet, using approximately 1 tablespoon for 8 servings, and heat it up with a medium-high flame. When the oil seems warm, test it by dropping in one slice of a vegetable. If the oil sizzles, it is ready and the rest of the ingredients can be added.

Either add the different kinds of vegetables one by one, starting with those that take the longest time to cook and ending with the faster-cooking ones, or cut the vegetables so that they will cook at the same rate (soft vegetables in larger slices, tougher ones in thinner slices), and layer them from yin to yang (yin on the bottom).

After adding the vegetables, add a pinch or two of sea salt. Salt brings out the natural sweetness, draws out the water, and helps to soften the vegetables quicker (it has the opposite effect on grains and beans and is therefore added later on in their case). Gently stir from time to time (with a wooden spoon or cooking chopsticks) to prevent burning.

After about 5 minutes turn the flame to low, cover (unless working with really watery items such as Chinese cabbage or tofu), and simmer until the vegetables are soft. The time it takes depends on what is being cooked and the size of slices used. It may be necessary to add a little water to avoid burning, especially when cooking with something like burdock. Add a little soy sauce (and some grated ginger if desired) at the end for more flavor, and simmer another 2 to 3 minutes. Uncover and boil away any excess water if there is any.

Any vegetable can be sautéed (cut root vegetables into very thin slices or shavings), as can tofu and tempeh.

Kinpira Carrot and Burdock
(Kinpira is very strengthening and can be used once or twice a week. While generally made with oil, the dish can also be made using the water-sautéing technique described above.)

1 cup shaved burdock
2 cups shaved carrots
Dark sesame oil (optional)
1 pinch sea salt
Tamari soy sauce to taste

Fig. 10   Burdock

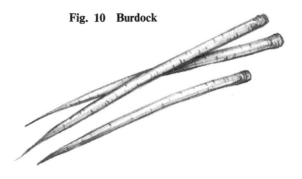

½ tsp. juice of grated ginger (optional)
Water, if needed to prevent burning
A few parsley sprigs

Lightly brush sesame oil in a skillet and heat. Place burdock
and carrots into the skillet and add a pinch of sea salt. Sauté
for 2 to 3 minutes. Add water to lightly cover the bottom of
the skillet. Cover and cook until the vegetables are 80 percent
done. Add several drops of tamari soy sauce, cover, and cook
for several minutes more until the vegetables become tender.
Remove the cover and cook until the excess liquid is absorbed.
Onions, turnips, and lotus root can be substituted or used
together with carrots and burdock.

Chinese Style Vegetables

½ Chinese cabbage
2 stalks celery
2 carrots
3 shiitake mushrooms
5 scallions
1 pinch sea salt
¼ tsp. sesame oil
Tamari soy sauce
2 Tbsps. kuzu
1½ cups water

Cut the cabbage into 1½-inch diagonal slices. Slice the celery
into 1½-inch, thin diagonal slices, and cut the scallions into
1½-inch diagonal pieces, separating the white bottom from the
greens. Cut the carrots in half lengthwise and then in thin
1½-inch-long diagonal slices. Soak the shiitake mushrooms
until tender and slice thin.

Warm a skillet on medium heat, add oil, and when the oil is
hot, add the scallion bottoms and the shiitake mushrooms.
Add salt and sauté for a few minutes, stirring as necessary to
prevent sticking. Add the carrots, stir, cover pan and reduce
the heat to medium-low. When the carrots have just begun to
soften (just a minute or two), add celery. After a few more
minutes add the Chinese cabbage and scallion greens.

Continue to cook until all the vegetables are cooked through,
but still slightly crunchy. Remove vegetables and place in
a serving dish. Dissolve kuzu in a small amount of cold water.
Add water and kuzu to the skillet and stir constantly while
bringing it to a boil. Season with tamari soy sauce and cook
for a few minutes more. Pour over vegetables. Grated ginger

and/or toasted sesame seeds can be added at the end of cooking.

Sautéed Mustard Greens

> **1 bunch fresh mustard greens**
> **$\frac{1}{8}$ tsp. sesame oil or water**
> **$\frac{1}{2}$ tsp. tamari soy sauce or to taste**
> **1 tsp. grated ginger**

Carefully wash greens and cut to desired shape. Warm a skillet on medium heat and add oil. When oil is hot, add the greens, stir and cover. Cook for about 3 minutes, or until the greens are tender. (Stir once or twice to ensure even cooking.) Remove pan from heat, and mix in tamari soy sauce and ginger. Serves 4 to 6.

4. *Pressure-cooking:* Pressure-cooking is a good way to prepare big chunks of root vegetables and squash (but don't cook greens this way). Use this style as often as desired as long as fresher vegetables such as salad and boiled or steamed greens are included to balance the pressure-cooking used for grains and beans. After the pressure comes up, carrots and onions may be done in 5 minutes, and big chunks of lotus root and burdock in 15 to 20 minutes.

After putting ingredients into the pressure cooker, add enough water to just cover the bottom of the pot (approximately $\frac{1}{2}$ to 1 inch). Add salt, cover, and bring to pressure over a medium-high flame. When pressure is up, turn the flame to low and simmer until done. Rinse the pot under cold water to bring the pressure down quickly, if desired, being careful not to uncover the pot until the pressure is completely down.

Pressure-cooked Squash

> **1 buttercup squash or Hokkaido pumpkin**
> **1 pinch sea salt**

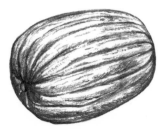

Fig. 11 Hokkaido Pumpkin

Enough water to cover the bottom of the pot

Scrub the dirt off the squash with a vegetable brush. Slice off
any crusty, flesh-colored growths on the skin. Cut the squash
open and remove the seeds. (These can be used for compost,
dried and planted in the spring, or toasted and eaten as
a snack.) Slice the squash into big, 1½- to 2-inch chunks, and
place them in the pressure cooker. Cover and follow the
preceeding directions, cooking the squash for about 10 minutes after the pressure comes up. Serves 4.

5. *Steaming:* Steaming can be used often. To steam, put ½ to
1 inch of cold water in the bottom of a pot, insert a steamer,
place vegetables inside, with a pinch of sea salt if desired, cover,
and bring the water to a boil. Then steam for 3 to 5 minutes
(greens should be steamed only about 3 minutes) or until the
vegetables are soft.

This method is good for any kind of vegetable and is a nice
variation on the boiling method. Be careful not to overcook the
vegetables. Remove them while they are still crisp and brightly
colored.

Steam each kind of vegetable separately unless they are to be
served mixed together and they take the same amount of time to
cook. In order for the vegetables to keep their bright color, run
them under cold water and don't cover them until they are cool.
The leftover water can be used as soup stock or sauce, as with
the boiling method. Steaming is also an excellent way to heat up
leftovers, especially grains.

Steamed Radishes and Greens

> **2 bunches radishes with greens intact**
> **1 pinch sea salt**
> **1 tsp. fresh toasted sesame seeds**

Bring a pot of water with a steamer basket in it to a full boil.
Meanwhile, wash radishes and slice them into ¼-inch-thick
rounds. Wash the greens well and cut them into 1-inch pieces.
Add the radishes to the steamer, placing the greens on top.
Add a pinch of sea salt and cook until the greens and radishes
are just tender, but not over-cooked. Remove from pot and
toss with sesame seeds, or arrange on a serving dish, and
sprinkle on the seeds.

Steamed Mixed Vegetables

4 cups broccoli flowers, approx.
1½ cups mung-bean sprouts, approx.
1 carrot, matchsticks
1 pinch sea salt

When the water is boiling, layer the carrots on the bottom, add the sprouts, and then the broccoli on top. Add a pinch of sea salt and cook for 3 to 5 minutes, or until the broccoli is just tender. Remove from the pot and serve as is, or tossed with a favorite dressing.

6. *Salad:* There are three types of salads:
   A. *Boiled salad:* Refer to the section on boiled vegetables for directions and an example. This can be eaten several times a week.

   B. *Pressed salad:* Pressed salad can generally be eaten every two or three days. The vegetables are raw but pressing them with salt helps to yangize them.
      To prepare, cut vegetables into very thin slices, or shred them, and put them in a pickle press with sea salt for one or more hours. Drain off the excess water, wash off the excess salt, and serve. To prepare without a pickle press, put vegetables in a bowl and cover them with a plate. Put a rock or some kind of weight (such as a large glass jar filled with water) on top of the plate and press.

Daikon Salad

4 cups daikon cut into very thin matchsticks
1½–2 tsp. sea salt

Mix ingredients thoroughly, rubbing salt into daikon. Press for

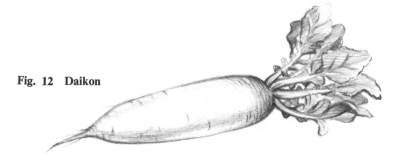

Fig. 12 Daikon

2 to 3 hours. If daikon is too salty, rinse with cold water before serving.

Cabbage Salad

$\frac{1}{2}$ **green cabbage**
$\frac{1}{4}$ **red cabbage**
1 onion
1$\frac{1}{2}$–2 Tbsps. umeboshi vinegar

Slice cabbages very thin. (You could also grate or shred them.) Slice onion very thin. Mix ingredients thoroughly with umeboshi vinegar and press for 1$\frac{1}{2}$ to 2 hours. Quickly rinse before serving if desired. Leftover salad can be pressed overnight for a quick pickle for the next evening's meal.

Pressed Salad

2 cups Chinese cabbage, finely shredded
$\frac{1}{4}$ **cup celery, sliced thinly on the diagonal**
$\frac{1}{2}$ **cup red radishes, thinly sliced**
1 tsp. sea salt

Place all vegetables in a pickle press. Add the sea salt and mix thoroughly. Apply pressure. Press 1$\frac{1}{2}$ to 2 hours. Drain off the juice which rises to the surface of the press.

C. Raw salad: Those with a more yin condition can have much less raw salad or avoid it altogether until their condition becomes more balanced. Normally, salad is eaten once or twice a week and those with a more yang condition could eat it frequently in the hot summer months if desired.

Use the usual salad vegetables such as lettuce, cucumbers, sprouts, carrots, onions, celery, parsley, cabbage, and so on, but avoid peppers, potatoes, tomatoes, eggplants, and mushrooms. Suggestions for additional ingredients include roasted sesame and pumpkin seeds, wholewheat bread croutons, cooked chick-peas, pinto beans, rice, bulgur, couscous, noodles, macaroni, wakame, dried dulse, and cooked hijiki, arame, tofu, tempeh and seitan. Of course, combinations have to be tasteful. Obviously, not all of these ingredients are compatible.

Wakame Salad

1 cup wakame (Wash, soak 10 minutes, boil 2–3 minutes, rinse in cold water, drain, and slice into 1" pieces.)

½ head iceburg lettuce, cut into bite-sized pieces
1 cucumber, sliced into thin rounds
1 Tbsp. umeboshi paste

Peel cucumber if it is waxed. Cut off the ends and dip them in sea salt. Rub each end piece in a circular motion against the end it was cut from. This helps draw out bitterness from the cucumber. Rinse off sea salt and slice cucumber. Mix wakame, umeboshi paste, lettuce, and cucumber. Serves 5.

Tossed Salad

1 head leafy green lettuce
1 cup alfalfa sprouts
½ cup carrot, cut into very thin matchsticks
1 red onion, sliced into thin rounds
½ pkg. tempeh, cut into cubes, deep-fried or pan-fried, and
    simmered in kombu stock with tamari soy sauce for ½ hour
1 recipe *Tamari, Ginger, Vinegar Dressing*

Wash lettuce, drain, and cut into bite-sized pieces. Toss all ingredients or arrange artfully on a serving platter. Serve the dressing on the side.

7. *Baking:* Baking foods takes a longer time but it gives strength and extra flavor. It is best to bake once in a while for variety rather than on a daily basis. The method is especially appropriate to the fall and winter seasons as it is a more yang cooking style, and is most suitable to root or round vegetables, such as winter squash. Greens should never be baked.

Baking can be done with or without oil, using a casserole dish or a cookie sheet covered with foil. If the vegetables are fresh and juicy, it may not be necessary to add water, especially if the sheet or dish is oiled and well-covered. If no oil is used, add just enough water to cover the cooking surface. More water may be needed if the vegetables are tough or a bit dried out. Adding a pinch of salt helps to draw out water from the vegetables.

The vegetables should be cooked at 350° to 375°F. for approximately 45 to 50 minutes, or until they are soft.

Squash can be baked whole and uncovered, on an oiled cookie sheet, with a stuffing, or sliced in halves or chunks. If halved, place the halves on a cookie sheet uncovered, with the inside facing down.

Baked Stuffed Squash

1–2 acorn squash

1 cup millet, pressure-cooked with 1½ cups spring water for
15 minutes, or boiled for 25 minutes with 2 cups water
¼ cup onions, diced
¼ cup carrots, diced
⅛ cup celery, diced
1 sliced mushroom
¾–1 cup chopped seitan

Combine the millet, onions, carrots, celery, mushroom, and seitan. Cut the tops off the squash and scoop out the seeds. Fill the squash with the millet mixture (if it is very dry, moisten this mixture with about ½ cup of seitan juice or spring water). Place the squash in a baking dish in which a small amount of spring water has been added. Cover the dish with foil and bake at 350°F. approximately 35 to 40 minutes or until the squash is tender.

Variations: For more ideas see *Baked Kombu and Vegetables* in the *Sea Vegetable* chapter. Tempeh, tofu, seitan, or fu could also be baked with vegetables.

Corn on the cob can also be baked; leave the inner husk on, rinse with cold water, leaving the corn dripping wet, and place in a 375°F. oven for about 30 minutes, or until done.

Yellow squash can also be baked as you would winter squash, reducing the cooking time.

8. *Pickles:* Pickles are an extremely important addition to the diet. Have a small amount on the side at every meal or at least once a day, and eat them with grains. They aid in digestion, strengthen the intestinal flora, stimulate appetite, and add zest to the meal. If the pickles are very salty, rinse them quickly before serving or, if necessary, soak them in cold water for 5 minutes.

Always use fresh, firm, and crisp vegetables for making pickles. Also, it is imperative that the vegetables, containers, and anything else used for pickling, be thoroughly cleaned. This is done to prevent any unknown substances interacting with the pickling process. For tougher vegetables, it is helpful to quickly blanch them in boiling water before pickling them.

Pickling time ranges from a couple of hours to several months. The main factors influencing pickling time are the size of vegetables and the amount of salt used. Small, thinly sliced pieces can be pickled very quickly whereas large, thick, or whole pieces take a long time. Long-time pickling requires more salt to prevent spoiling. Vegetables can be dipped in hot boiling water before pickling, if desired, especially with largely sliced and/or hard vegetables. This removes the raw flavor and brings out a sweeter taste.

Experimentation may be needed to get the feel of the right amount of salt to use. If the vegetables spoil before they pickle, and/or not much water comes out (for methods that require that it does), then there is not enough salt. If too much salt is added, the pickles will become too salty and any other flavor that the vegetables may have had will be covered up. To remove excess salt, rinse or soak pickles for a little while before serving them.

If mold starts to form anywhere, remove it immediately so that the rest of the contents will not be affected.

Cover the container with a cheesecloth. This helps to keep dirt and dust out of the pickles while letting the air circulate and enabling the vegetables to breathe. (Do not cover with an airtight lid.)

There are four main types of pickling methods that we usually use.

1. *Pressed pickles:* Pressed pickles can be made quickly, in a couple of hours, or over several weeks.

   A. *Quick pickles:* When pickling for a few hours up to a day or two, a pickle press can be used. But since most presses are made of plastic, it is not safe to use them for a longer period of time as the poisonous toxic substances in them will start to seep into the vegetables. An alternative is to take a small glass bowl and find a saucer that fits into it. It should cover the inside as much as possible but still remain loose so that water can escape over the sides. For a weight, use a glass jar full of water, grains, or beans, or some clean stones.

   Soft, watery vegetables like thinly sliced cucumbers and very thin matchstick daikon strips can be done in 2 to 3 hours. Other pickles can be made in the morning and be either eaten for dinner or left for 2 to 3 days longer. Some (like harder, less watery vegetables like turnips) may need the extra days. Again, pickling time depends on the size and moisture content of the pieces.

   Vegetables have to be cut into really thin slices or shredded for quick pickling. (An exception is mustard greens which can be made whole and cut when ready to serve. Mix the salt in really well and wait 2 to 3 days.) Chinese cabbage, red and white cabbage, daikon and its greens, turnip and its greens, celery, radishes, onions, cucumbers, and bok choy are good to use. For best results, use only one kind of vegetable at a time. Add a strip of kombu (perhaps 3 to 6 inches long for two cups of vegetables) for extra minerals and a different flavor. Soak the kombu until it is soft, slice it into thin strips, and put it underneath the vegetables. Grated ginger can be added if desired. For 2 cups of vegetables add about 1 to 2 teaspoons of salt. Mix them together thoroughly. The salt can be substituted with 2 to 4 tablespoons of umeboshi vinegar, paste, or plums and/or shiso leaves. You can also use 2 to 4 tablespoons of soy sauce. Water will start to rise above the saucer or pressure plate. If there is a lot, remove a little, but always leave some of it covering the plate. Cover with a cheesecloth (not necessary if using a press, of course) and wait till it is all done.

Onion Pickles

2 cups thinly sliced onions
2–4 Tbsp. tamari soy sauce

Pickle the onions in soy sauce following the above directions. If the onions were cut thinly, they will be done in 2 hours. You can also eat them the next day.

B. *Longer-time pressed pickles:* A wooden keg or ceramic crock are good containers to use for this. A heavy stone or large jar filled with water is placed on top of a plate or a wooden disc, which fits inside, for pressure. Cover the whole thing with a cheesecloth and place in a cool, dark place. Check regularly for mold and remove it immediately if any appears. Sauerkraut is made this way. Below is a sample recipe.

Pressed Daikon Pickles

4–5 daikon radish
½ cup sea salt

Wash, dry completely and cut the daikon into several lengthwise strips. Place a layer of salt in a crock or wooden keg. Then add a layer of daikon. Then a layer of salt. Alternate until all the daikon is used. Salt should be the last layer. Place a weight on top, cover with a cheesecloth, and press for 1 to 2 weeks. Chinese cabbage, carrots, turnips, daikon greens, and so on can all be pickled this way.

2. *Brine pickles:* To make brine pickles, tightly stuff some vege-

tables into a glass jar. Boil some kind of a brine mixture (see below), let it cool, and then pour it into the jar, filling it up. Cover the top with cheesecloth which is fastened down with a rubber band, and pickle for several days. When done, store pickles in a refrigerator. This is how dill pickles are made. A variety of vegetables can be used, including cucumbers, onions, turnips, rutabagas, daikon, carrots, broccoli, cauliflower, cabbages, greens, and so on.

There are several kinds of brine that can be used, examples of which are presented below. A soup stock can be used if desired. For extra flavor, add ginger, kombu, shiitake mushrooms, lemon juice and rinds, shiso leaves, grated raw apple, and so on. Some *ame* rice syrup can be boiled and dissolved into the brine, especially in the case of tamari-based pickles, as it gives a delicious sweet taste.

Onion Cucumber Pickles (Salt-based Brine)

3 lbs. pickling cucumbers
2 onions, quartered
12 cups spring water
$\frac{1}{4}$–$\frac{1}{3}$ cup sea salt

Bring water and salt to a boil. Turn flame to medium-low and simmer until all the salt has dissolved. Allow this mixture to cool. Wash and place cucumbers and onions into a large glass jar or crock. Pour the cooled brine in, filling the container to the top. Cover with a cheesecloth and keep in a cool, dark place for 5 to 10 days. When pickles are done, store them in the refrigerator.

Turnip Pickles

4 turnips, sliced very thinly, lengthwise
1$\frac{1}{2}$ tsps. sea salt
2 tsps. chopped lemon peel

Mix all ingredients together by hand. Place the turnips in a bowl, cover, and leave overnight. Rinse the pickles before eating them. These can be refrigerated for up to one week.

Cauliflower and Radish Pickles (Umeboshi-based Brine)

Enough cauliflower to fill a glass quart jar
5 radishes, cut in half
2 cups water
1 cup umeboshi vinegar

5 shiso leaves

Place cauliflower and radishes into a jar. Mix the water, umeboshi vinegar, and shiso leaves together and pour over vegetables. Cover with a cheesecloth and let set for 3 to 4 days.

3. *Miso pickles:* Miso pickles are especially helpful for recovering
good digestive strength. They are simple to make. Just quickly
blanch vegetables in boiling water, then submerge and sur-
round them totally in miso. This is used for root vegetables
such as carrots, burdock, daikon, turnips, parsnips, and ginger.
Broccoli stems make great pickles as well. Greens are too
watery.

The vegetables have to be dried out until they can be bent
like rubber before being added to the miso. Otherwise, the
miso will get too watery and the pickling won't work.

Pickling time depends on the vegetables being used and the
size of the slices. Very thin ones can pickle in 3 to 4 days, up
to a week. Whole vegetables with slits in their sides can take
1 to 2 weeks, thick slices about 3 months, and whole vegetables (unslitted) can be left in the miso up to a year. Just
make sure they are totally submerged (top, bottom, and sides).
Pressure is not needed when making miso pickles.

When the pickles are done, just take them out, rinse them
off, slice, and eat them.

Broccoli Stem Miso Pickles

Broccoli stems
A container of miso

Peel leftover broccoli stems unless the skins are soft, quickly
blanch them in boiling water, and submerge them into the
miso for 1 to 2 weeks, depending on how thick they are. You
can leave the skins on if you like. The pickling time will be

Fig. 13 Broccoli

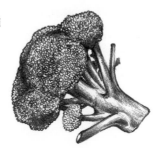

much longer then, maybe a month or more. Cover with a cheesecloth and keep in a cool, dark place until they are done.

4. *Bran pickles:* Bran pickling uses a mixture of bran (rice or wheat) or rice flour, and sea salt. Like miso pickles, bran pickles are especially good for weak intestines.

Quickly dry-roast the bran or flour in a skillet over a medium-low flame until a nutty fragrance is emitted. Remove from the skillet and allow it to cool.

Firm, root vegetables pickle best, but you can also use greens. The vegetables should all be dried before you use them. A few hours under the sun works nicely. Daikon, carrots, and parsnips are best when dried longer (several days), until they bend like rubber.

A ceramic crock or wooden keg again are the best containers to use. Cover the pickles with a cheesecloth and keep in a cool, dark place.

There are two ways to make bran pickles.

A. *Bran pickles A:* Boil some salt and water, let it cool off, place in a crock or keg, and thoroughly mix in the roasted bran or flour to form a paste. Take your dried vegetables and totally submerge them into this paste making sure that the vegetables are not touching each other. Pack this whole thing down until it is firm and solid. Cover with a cheesecloth.

If you slice the vegetables into fairly small pieces they will be done in a week or two. You can also leave them whole. Whole root vegetables can take as long as 3 to 5 months to pickle. Add more salt if you want to pickle for a long time. (Whole leaves take only a couple of weeks.)

As you remove your finished pickles, you can keep adding new vegetables. When you do, add more bran and salt. Mix the paste once in a while. If kept well, you can use this paste for years as you add and subtract vegetables from it.

Short-Time Paste Proportions (1–2 Weeks)

10–12 cups bran or rice flour
$\frac{1}{8}$–$\frac{1}{4}$ cup sea salt
3–5 cups water

Longer-Time Paste Proportions (Up to 3–5 Months)

10–12 cups bran or rice flour

1½–2 cups sea salt
3–5 cups water

B. *Bran pickles B:* This method is made by alternating
layers of vegetables with layers of the bran and sea salt mixture.
   Mix roasted bran with sea salt and cover the bottom of
a crock or keg. Then, add a layer of dried vegetables. Add
another layer of bran and salt. Keep alternating. The last
layer should be bran. Insert a plate or a wooden disc into the
crock on top of the mixture, place a heavy weight on top of
the plate, and press the whole thing. The plate or disc should
be loose fitting but wide enough to cover the contents as much
as possible. A clean stone or a jar filled with water can be used
as a weight. Cover with a cheesecloth and put in a cool, dark
place. When water begins to rise, lighten the weight. When
pickles are done, rinse off the bran, slice, and eat.
   Just as in *Bran pickles A*, you can either slice the vegetables
into fairly small pieces or leave them whole. As before, whole
pieces take a much longer time to pickle and require more salt.

● **Short-Time Proportions (1–2 Weeks)**

10–12 cups bran or rice flour
⅛–¼ cups sea salt

● **Longer-Time Proportions (3–5 Months)**

10–12 cups bran or rice flour
1½–2 cups sea salt

Chinese Cabbage Bran Pickles

2 heads Chinese cabbage
Bran & salt using shorter-time proportions

Separate the individual leaves from the body of the cabbage.
Dry the leaves for two days, preferably under the sun. Make
alternating layers of cabbage with sea salt (the bottom and top
layers should be salt) and place a plate and heavy weight on
top. Water should rise to the level of the plate in 10 hours.
If not, add more weight and/or a little more salt.
   When the water has risen, drain it out thoroughly. Then
relayer the cabbage alternating it with the bran. (The bottom
and top layers should be bran.) Replace the weight.

The pickles should be ready in a week. When done, wash out the bran, slice, and serve. (The reason for draining out the water first is to produce a less salty and more sweet-tasting pickle. Also, the Chinese cabbage is a pretty watery vegetable. Other vegetables can be layered in one step, using the bran the first time around, as mentioned before this recipe.)

11. Sea Vegetables ━━━━━━━━

Sea vegetables are an important and integral part of the macrobiotic diet. They help purify and strengthen the bloodstream and strengthen the intestines, digestive system, liver, pancreas, sexual organs, and enhance mental clarity and awareness. They also help promote beautiful skin and hair. Sea vegetables can be consumed every day in some form, whatever one's condition. They supply calcium, iron, protein, iodine, and vitamins A, B$_{12}$, and C, as well as various other minerals.

Many people used to (and some still do) cringe at the thought of eating sea vegetables, and considered it an esoteric Oriental food. However, sea vegetables were consumed traditionally by people all over the world including the Celtics, Vikings, Russians, coastal Africans, Mediterranean peoples, North and South American Indians, native Australians, and the early New England settlers (dulse and kombu in their case), as well as people in the Far East. Some varieties may take a while to acquire a taste for, but it is well worth the effort for all the benefits that they bestow.

Sea vegetables are purchased dried (from natural food stores) and can be kept for quite a while before using. They are easily stored. Any shady, dry place will do.

Several varieties of sea vegetables are now available. Kombu is more tough and may take several hours of cooking, unless pressure-cooked, to completely soften. Dulse, on the other hand, can be eaten raw, or like nori, just toasted for a few seconds.

Wash sea vegetables very quickly to retain as much of their nutrients as possible. Submerge hijiki, wakame, and arame in water, rinse off any dust that floats to the top, and lift them out of the water, leaving behind any sand or stones that sit at the bottom. (Arame will probably be pretty clean already as it has been shredded.)

To clean kombu, brush off any dirt or dust with a dry or damp towel. Leave the white-colored substance (which consists of salt and complex sugars) on the surface of the kombu, as it contributes to the flavor and nutritional value. Dulse does not need to be washed in water, but check it very carefully for hidden shells, stones, and tiny fish. Nori and agar-agar should not be washed.

1. *Arame and hijiki:*   Arame comes shredded and has a very delicious but mild flavor. Hijiki is naturally stringy and looks like a thicker, darker arame. It also has a richer taste. Hijiki should be soaked for 3 to 5 minutes until it expands a bit. Remember that it finally

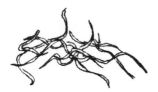
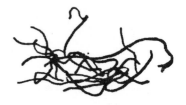

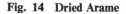

Fig. 14   Dried Arame   Fig. 15   Dried Hijiki

becomes 3 to 5 times larger, so be careful not to use more than you need. It is not necessary to soak arame, just quickly rinse it once in cold water.

Arame and hijiki are cooked the same way, though hijiki takes a longer time, and one can be substituted for the other. They combine really well with root vegetables or with seitan, tofu, tempeh, and fresh corn, as well as other ingredients. They are generally sautéed or just simmered with a small amount of water. It is nice occasionally to sauté the vegetables first before adding the sea vegetable.

2. *Kombu:* Kombu comes in thick, flat strips which may be anywhere from 3 to 18 inches long. There are recipes throughout this cookbook using kombu, as it enhances the flavor of grains, beans, and vegetable dishes, helping them to soften and/or effectively combining and synthesizing all the ingredients into a whole. It also makes an excellent soup stock. (See *Soup* chapter.) In many cases, kombu is used as an accessory to other ingredients in a dish, but it can be used as a vegetable in its own right. Its texture tends to be tough, so pressure-cooking is often the preferred cooking method, although it can also be boiled.

Kombu needs to be soaked before slicing. It doubles in size, so be careful how much is used. Soak only until it becomes soft

Fig. 16   Kombu

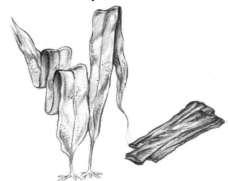

enough to cut. Otherwise, it becomes slippery and slicing will be difficult.

3. *Wakame:* Wakame is a thin, leafy type of sea vegetable and cooks quickly. It can be used in any recipe that calls for kombu. As is kombu, wakame is excellent in grains, beans, vegetable dishes, and soups.

    Wakame should be soaked before being sliced. If the soaking water is a bit salty, save it for soups, grains, or bean dishes, where it will be more diluted. Or, to use some of the flavor that went into the liquid for the wakame dish, combine a portion of it with fresh water.

    The vein portion takes a longer time to cook. Slice that part fairly thin so that it will be finished when the softer leafy sections (which should be sliced into larger pieces) are.

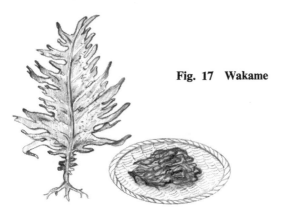

Fig. 17 Wakame

4. *Nori:* Nori comes in thin, flat, paper-like sheets. No washing, soaking, or cooking is required except to lightly toast it over an open flame for a few seconds. In Japan it is used to garnish noodles, grains, and vegetables, and as a wrapping for sushi and rice balls, among other things.

Fig. 18 Nori

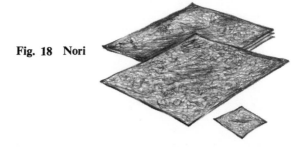

Toast the nori by waving the dull side over the flame on an open gas burner. After toasting the sheets, they can be torn or cut with scissors, or left whole. Very small pieces or slivers make a good decorative garnish on top of noodles, grains, vegetables, and so on. One-eighth of a sheet is a nice size for covering and picking up small pieces of grains or vegetables. Two pieces (a quarter sheet) are used to wrap a rice ball.

6. *Sea palm:*   Sea palm is a beautiful, green sea vegetable which grows on the rocks of the Pacific coast. It comes in long fronds and can be cleaned, then soaked as is done for hijiki. Sea palm can also be a little salty, so you may choose not to use the soaking water. Cook for 30 to 45 minutes.

5. *Dulse:*   Dulse can be added raw or slightly toasted to soups, salads, and vegetable, grain, and bean dishes, at the very end of preparation, for extra flavor. It can also be lightly toasted by itself, crumbled and used as a condiment.

6. *Agar-agar:*   Agar-agar is used as a jelling agent for kantens and aspics. It can be purchased in the form of bars or powder, and comes with cooking instructions enclosed. (See *Desserts* section for kanten recipes.)

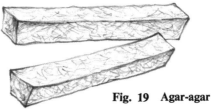

Fig. 19   Agar-agar

Arame with Sweet Corn

>   **1 oz. dried arame**
>   **1 cup onions, sliced in half-moons**
>   **Water**
>   **1–3 Tbsps. tamari soy sauce**
>   **2 cups fresh, sweet corn kernels**
>   ***Optional:*   1 tsp. dark sesame oil**

Clean arame and put it in a strainer to drain. Heat oil in a frying pan. (If you do not wish to use oil, use a small amount of water here.) Sauté the onions for 1 to 2 minutes, stirring to ensure even cooking. Add the arame on top and enough water to just cover the onions. Add a little tamari soy sauce. Cover and bring to a boil, then turn the flame to medium-low, and simmer for about 20 minutes. Add the corn and a little more tamari to taste. Simmer for 10 to 15 minutes more, or until liquid has evaporated.

Arame with Dried Tofu and Carrots

> **1 oz. dried arame**
> **2 pieces dried tofu, soaked and cubed**
> **Spring water**
> **1 cup carrots, cut into matchsticks**
> **2 tsps. tamari soy sauce**
> **$\frac{1}{2}$ Tbsp. mirin**

Wash the arame and drain in a colander. Heat enough spring water to just cover the bottom of a skillet. Add the arame and carrots and sauté 1 to 2 minutes.

Add the dried tofu and enough water to cover the arame and carrots. Add a little tamari soy sauce. Bring to a boil, cover, and reduce the heat to low. Simmer for 40 to 45 minutes. Season with a little more tamari soy sauce and the mirin, and simmer for 10 to 15 minutes longer. When nearly all the liquid has evaporated, mix and serve.

Hijiki with Carrots and Lotus Root

> **1 oz. hijiki**
> **1 cup carrots, cut into thin matchsticks**
> **$\frac{3}{4}$ cup lotus root, sliced into thin half-moons**
> **Water**
> **Tamari soy sauce**
> *Optional:* **$\frac{1}{4}$ tsp. dark sesame oil**

Wash and drain hijiki. (If it is still tough, it can be soaked for 3 to 5 minutes. The soaking water can be used in cooking if it is not too salty.) Heat a skillet with a small amount of oil (you can just brush the bottom) or water. Sauté the hijiki and carrots for 2 to 3 minutes. Add water to half the height of the ingredients. Layer lotus root on top and add a small amount of tamari soy sauce. Cover, bring to a boil, and simmer for 35 to 40 minutes. Add more tamari to taste if desired, and continue to cook for 20 minutes more or until liquid evaporates.

Hijiki with Sesame Seeds

> **1 oz. hijiki**
> **Tamari soy sauce**

Water
¼ cup toasted sesame seeds
½ tsp. grated ginger

Wash hijiki and soak it for 3 to 5 minutes if tough. (Use this soaking water if it is not too salty.) Place hijiki in a skillet and add water to half the height of the sea vegetable. Add a small amount of tamari soy sauce, cover, bring to a boil, and simmer for 45 to 55 minutes, or until water has evaporated. Mix in grated ginger and toasted sesame seeds. Serve.

Variations: As you can see, hijiki and arame can be cooked in the same manner, hijiki taking a little longer than arame. Though these sea vegetables are usually sautéed (with or without oil), you can also just simmer them. Hijiki and arame can be substituted for each other in most any recipe, adjusting the cooking times. Other variations include: Adding dried daikon, fresh tofu, tempeh, as well as deep-fried or pan-fried tofu or tempeh. Scallions, ginger, or toasted seeds can be added at the end of cooking. A little rice vinegar (for those with a more yang condition) can also be added toward the end of cooking for a delicious flavor.

Baked Kombu and Vegetables

1 strip kombu, 3″
2 onions, peeled and quartered
2 carrots, cut into triangular shapes
½ cabbage, sliced into ½″ strips
½ cup spring water
1½ Tbsps. tamari soy sauce

Wash and soak the kombu and put it in a baking dish. Arrange the onions in one side of the dish, the carrots in the center, and the cabbage at the other side, being sure to keep the vegetables separated. Pour the water into a dish and add the tamari soy sauce. Cover and bake in a preheated 375°F. oven for 30 to 40 minutes, or until all the ingredients are tender.

Variations: Many different vegetables can be used in this dish. For a sweet variation, try winter squash with onions. Burdock, parsnips, lotus root, daikon, celery, Brussels sprouts, rutabaga, and cauliflower can also be cooked this way.

Wakame can be used instead of kombu, and sea salt can be used with or instead of tamari soy sauce. Grated ginger, chopped scallions, parsley, or chives can be used as a garnish.

Kombu and Dried Daikon

2 3″-strips kombu
½ cup dried daikon, soaked and sliced
Vegetable soaking water
Tamari soy sauce

Wash, soak, and thinly slice the kombu. Put the kombu in a pot and place the dried daikon on top. Add the soaking water to just cover and bring to a boil. Cover and turn the heat to low. Simmer for 40 to 45 minutes, or until the kombu is very soft. Season with a little tamari soy sauce to taste and simmer until the remaining liquid has almost evaporated.

Variations: Soaked and sliced shiitake mushrooms (3 to 4) can be cooked with daikon and kombu. (This is helpful for those with a more yang condition.)

Wakame and Onions

1 oz. dried wakame
3 small onions, sliced
Tamari soy sauce, about 1–2 tsp.

Wash, soak, and slice the wakame into 1-inch pieces. Put the wakame and onions in a pot, side by side. Add enough soaking water to almost cover the sea vegetable. Bring to a boil, reduce heat to low, and simmer for 30 minutes, or until tender. Some varieties take longer to cook than others. Add tamari soy sauce to taste and cook for 10 to 15 minutes longer.

Wakame, Broccoli, and Onions

1 cup washed, soaked and sliced wakame
6 broccoli flowerets
1 onion, sliced into thin half-moons
Water
A handful of toasted sesame seeds
Tamari soy sauce
***Optional:* Rice vinegar**

Slice the vein portion of the wakame into smaller pieces than the soft leaf part. Bring water to a boil and boil the broccoli until bright green and tender. Remove and drain in a colander. Boil onions until translucent, remove, and drain. Blanch wakame in boiling water, remove, and drain. Arrange the three vegetables attractively on a serving dish. Make a dressing with tamari *soy sauce*, vinegar, seeds, and water, and pour on top of vegetables. (This can also be used as a dipping sauce.)

Norimaki (Sushi)
(Sushi rolls are handy as appetizers, snacks, and for traveling, and have a very decorative appearance.)

$1\frac{1}{2}$ cups cooked short-grain (sticks best) brown rice
1 sheet nori
1 carrot, cut into several lengthwise strips
2–3 uncut (except for the roots) scallions
1″ boiling water in a pot
$\frac{1}{4}$–$\frac{1}{2}$ tsp. umeboshi paste
1 pinch sea salt

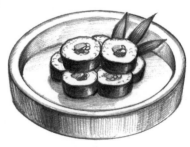

Fig. 20   Sushi

Add a pinch of salt (for brighter vegetable colors) to the boiling water and cook the carrot strips until they are soft. Remove the strips and let them drain. Next, boil the scallions (cut off the roots) for just a second, but not until they loose the bright green color, then remove and drain them.

Meanwhile, toast a sheet of nori by passing it over an open flame (on the dull side only for easier rolling) until it is green but not so much that it is overly crisp and crinkly.

Place a sushi mat on a cutting board, and lay the sheet of nori on top of it. The halfway fold of the nori should be horizontal to the cook. With wet hands, evenly press a $\frac{1}{4}$-inch layer of rice onto the nori, leaving $\frac{1}{2}$ to $\frac{3}{4}$ inch of the top edge (the side away from one) and $\frac{1}{4}$ inch of the bottom edge uncovered. Then, make a horizontal indentation in the rice 1 inch up from the bottom of the nori and spread the umeboshi paste inside the length of it. Then press 1 to 3 carrot strips and the scallions (again horizontally) on top of the paste.

Next, slowly roll the mat and its contents upwards, pressing firmly upon the rice and other ingredients. Try to tuck the vegetables underneath while rolling. Wet the top edge of the uncovered nori (to help in sealing) and complete the roll.

With dry hands, place the roll with the sealed edge underneath, wet a vegetable knife (to prevent the rice from sticking to it for smooth, easy cutting), and slowly, carefully and firmly cut the roll into 1-inch slices. Place the slices onto a plate with the inside turned upward to show their beautiful design, then decorate, and serve. Makes 5 pieces.

Dulse, Carrots, and Celery

2 cups carrots, halved and sliced on a diagonal
1 cup celery sliced on a diagonal
$\frac{1}{2}$ oz. dried dulse
Water

Pour a little water into a pot and bring to a boil. Reduce the heat to medium-low. Add the carrots and cook until tender. Remove, and put carrots in a bowl. Add the celery to the boiling water and simmer until just tender. Wash the dulse and cut it into small pieces. Remove celery, drain, and mix with carrots and dulse.

Azuki Bean Aspic

1 cup azuki beans
$\frac{1}{8}$ cup raisins
4 cups water
$\frac{1}{2}$ tsp. sea salt or 1 Tbsp. tamari soy sauce
1 bar agar-agar or equivalent in flakes or powder

Wash beans and combine them with the raisins in a pot. Add the water. Bring to a boil, reduce the heat to low, cover, and simmer until the beans are soft, about $1\frac{1}{2}$ hours. Quickly rinse the agar-agar bar and add to the beans. Add the seasoning. Thoroughly mix and cook for another 10 to 15 minutes. Pour into individual serving dishes or a large mold. Refrigerate until jelled. Serve cool.

Variations: Other good combinations are split peas and fresh peas; lentils and carrots; and carrots or squash and onions.

12. Seasonings and Condiments ━━━

Besides ingredients and cooking methods, seasonings and condiments play a vital part in the balancing of a meal. As with any other aspect of preparing foods, care must be taken to have enough variety. The chart below lists some of the condiments mentioned in this book. They are categorized into the five tastes. Making sure to use items from each column insures a well-rounded diet.

SOUR	BITTER	SWEET	PUNGENT	SALTY
Pickles	Gomashio	Miso	Ginger	Miso
Sauerkraut	Tekka	Amazaké	Scallions	Gomashio
Umeboshi	Green nori	Applesauce	Onions	Umeboshi
Shiso leaves	Parsley	Rice syrup	Grated daikon	Shiso leaves
Rice vinegar	Dandelion	Barley malt	Watercress	Shio kombu
Lemon	Wakame powder	Mirin		Wakame
	Mustard greens	Raisins		powder
	(pickled)			Tamari
				soy sauce
				Tekka

Seasonings: ━━━━━━━━━━━━━━━━━━━━━━━━━

1. *Sea salt:* Salt is one of the building blocks of life and we cannot survive without it. It is one of the basic ingredients of our blood and gives us vitality, strength, and mental clarity. Learning how to adjust salt intake and finding its balance with oil and water is an important part of mastering the art of cooking.

   Use only white unrefined sea salt. In commercial table salt, much of the valuable trace minerals have been removed. Sugar (dextrose), magnesium and sodium carbonate, and potassium iodine have been added in their place. Such salt depletes important minerals from the body and contributes to high blood pressure, heart problems, kidney disorders, and illness in general. Grey sea salt is also not recommended as it can cause excessive tightness in the body.

   The amount of salt that an individual needs depends on personal condition, age, activity level, and seasonal and other environmental factors. Physically active people, adults, persons with a more vegetarian-based history, and persons that live in a more wet, humid, and cold climate, can take more salt. (Babies should not take salt at all. It should be gradually introduced to their diet as they grow.) Individuals with a history of heavy meat consumption should carefully limit their salt intake and may even need to abstain for a short period of time. (These are the persons that benefit from vegetarian, raw food, and salt-free diets, which help to cleanse their bodies. However, after a while, salt and cooked foods should be reintroduced.)

Too much salt can cause hyperactivity, irritability, kidney problems, thirst and anger, among other things. Too little salt can cause poor circulation, mental lethargy, sleepiness, weakness, and so on. (Excess salt can also cause these symptoms at times.)

Meals should not be overwhelmingly salty. Salt should enhance and draw out the natural flavor and sweetness of foods, not cover them up. Generally, if, after meals, one becomes extremely thirsty or craves fatty, rich foods or strongly yin items such as sugar, ice cream, and so on, it is likely that an excess of salty (or hot) condiments and dishes have been consumed. Salt is very yang and attracts much yin, so too much makes it difficult to eat in a centered manner.

Plain salt is not recommended for use at the table. (An exception may be a small pinch on fresh fruits to draw out their sweetness.) It is too strong and difficult to assimilate in that form. Various condiments which substitute for salt—such as sea-vegetable powders or a mixture of salt and sesame seeds—are recommended. (See the *Condiments* section in this chapter.)

2. *Miso:* Miso is a paste made of fermented soybeans and sea salt which has been aged for a period of a few months to as much as three years or more. Miso only a few months old is light in color and contains less salt. If older, the color becomes a dark brown, and more salt is used to keep it going.

    The darker, longer-time miso is best for healing and is the kind that is assumed when using miso is recommended. The best miso is at least two summers old. There are three basic kinds now available in natural food stores. (Do not buy miso from Oriental food shops. It may be made without using a natural fermenting process, and also may contain chemicals and sugars.)

    A. *Hatcho miso:* Hatcho miso is 100 percent soybeans and is the darkest, most yang variety. It is especially recommended for the cold winter months.
    B. *Mugi miso:* Mugi miso contains barley, is the sweetest of the three, and can be used all year round. It also has medicinal properties.

C. *Genmai (brown rice) or Kome (white rice) miso:* These misos contain rice. They are lighter and are good for the summer though they can also be used year round. Use this variety less often than the first two.

The short-term miso comes in red, yellow, or white. It is sweet, good for summer use, and makes delicious sauces and spreads but does not have medicinal value.

Buying bulk miso is recommended over the packaged variety, especially when one is trying to heal oneself, as it is more alive. Before being packaged, miso has to be pasteurized, otherwise it will keep fermenting and may burst its container.

Keep the bulk miso in a cool, dark place, and stir it from time to time. (The short-term kind should be refrigerated.) If a white color starts to appear on the surface, mix it into the bulk of the miso. This substance is a natural bacterial growth and is not harmful. On the contrary, besides adding more minerals and flavor to the miso, it is a reassurance that the miso is organic and alive.

3. *Tamari soy sauce and/or shoyu:* Tamari soy sauce is a liquid by-product of the miso-making process. It contains fermented soybeans, water, sea salt, and sometimes a small amount of wheat. Be very careful to avoid commercial shoyu as it is artificially aged and is full of chemicals and coloring. To be on the safe side, purchase soy sauce from natural food stores instead of Oriental ones.

Tamari soy sauce can be added to just about any kind of dish for extra flavor. There are numerous recipes which use it throughout this book.

Like salt and miso, tamari soy sauce should always be cooked into foods, not added afterward at the table, as this can cause tightness, produce cravings for sweets, and disrupt digestion. Also, be careful not to take too much of it.

4. *Umeboshi plum, paste, and vinegar, and shiso-leaf pickle:* Umeboshi plums have very strong medicinal value. They purify the bloodstream, detoxify poisons, stimulate appetite, and at times can help to relieve stomachaches, nausea, and air sickness. (Take them along whenever traveling.) When someone is not feeling well, we separate the meat of the plums from the pit, grind it into a paste in a suribachi, or just chop it very finely, and add it to a thick kuzu drink (see *Special Needs* chapter), or serve it with rice cream.

Umeboshi plums have been pickled in sea salt and shiso leaves

(to give the plums their bright red color) for a year or more.
They can be added to just about any dish and may be used as
a substitute for salt, tamari soy sauce, or miso. One plum is a
delicious condiment with a bowl of rice or other grains. (See
Grains and Grain Products chapter for a rice ball recipe.)

Recently, umeboshi paste and umeboshi vinegar (leftover juice
from making these pickles) have become available. They are very
handy to cook with and can be added to various dishes. However,
they do not have the strong healing qualities of the plum. Therefore, when making *Special Needs* recipes or when trying to relieve
a stomachache (for instance) use the whole plum.

Pickled shiso leaves are also available by themselves. They can
be sliced and added to dishes in addition to, or as a substitute for,
salt. They are valuable when dried or baked and ground into
a powder for use as a condiment. In this form, they are helpful
for neutralizing strong chemicals in the system.

5. *Oil:* Vegetable oils, which are full of polyunsaturated fatty acids,
   are needed to build new cells and tissues, to keep warm, for
   vitamins A and E, to maintain proper metabolism, and to lubri-
   cate skin and hair, among other things. However, much of the oil
   we need is already found in grains, beans, and seeds, so the intake
   of extra oil can be kept to a minimum, especially during the
   initial few months of healing. A healthy person can have a small
   amount of extra oil nearly every day in a side dish of sautéed
   vegetables or in a sauce or dressing. Even then, one or two tablespoons are adequate to sauté enough vegetables and grains for
   a whole family. Also, deep-fried foods should not be consumed
   more than once a week.

   Choose unrefined and cold-pressed oils (meaning that the seeds
   have been pressed below the boiling point and filtered). Such oils
   have all their vitamins and nutrients intact, are rich in color,
   retain the flavor and taste of the original seeds, and are somewhat
   cloudy in appearance. Please avoid refined oils or oils that have
   been processed at a high temperature.

   Animals oils and fats should be totally avoided as they contain
   high levels of cholesterol which causes hardening of the arteries
   and heart disease, among other things.

   To digest more oily foods such as fried rice, accompany them
   with grated ginger, or grated, raw daikon, or plenty of chopped
   raw scallions.

   Keep oils in a tightly sealed container in a cool, dark place, or
   in the refrigerator.

   Sesame oil, especially the dark variety made from roasted seeds, is the most healthy oil to use as it is easiest to digest and more yang than other varieties. Pumpkin seed oil is an occasional variation, and is also more yang than other oils.

Corn oil (a lighter oil for pastries or pie crusts), safflower, sunflower, and olive oil may all be used occasionally once sound health is established. It is best to avoid them until then.

6. *Brown Rice Vinegar:* Brown rice vinegar is to be used occasionally. It is delicious in sushi, dressings, grain salads, and pickles.

7. *Mirin:* Mirin is a cooking wine made from sweet rice. It is delicious in sweet-and-sour sauces, as well as in beans, vegetables, noodle broths, dressings, and marinades. Use this occasionally; it may be avoided initially for several months.

8. *Ginger:* Ginger is a hot, pungent, and very delicious root which stimulates the appetite, and activates circulation.

   A small amount of grated ginger spices up grains, vegetables, and noodles. Extract the juice by squeezing the grated ginger. (The juice is stronger.) Ginger is taken raw or added at the very end of preparations.

9. *Rice syrup and barley malt:* These are the most healthy sweeteners that we use. They are the "honeys" of their respective grains, and are delicious in desserts or cooked in with azuki or black soybeans.

Condiments

Condiments, though we use them sparingly, are an indispensable part of macrobiotic eating. They add one or more of the following to a meal: color, extra variety and flavor, extra vitamins and minerals, appetite stimulation, balance, zest, and in some cases, medicinal value.

A small amount of various condiments may be used every day to accompany grains. They allow individuals to adjust their intake of salt, minerals, or oils to fit their personal needs. They are easy to overuse so be careful, especially when dealing with the saltier varieties such as gomashio or tekka.

Gomashio
(Gomashio, the most commonly used condiment in the Macrobiotic diet, is a perfect balance of salt and oil.)

14–16 Tbsps. black or white sesame seeds
1 level Tbsp. sea salt

Dry-roast sea salt in a skillet until it becomes shiny. (Roasting releases moisture in the salt and this helps to make a fluffier gomashio.) Place the roasted salt in a suribachi, and gently grind it to a fine powder.

Wash and rinse the sesame seeds and drain them in a fine wire-mesh strainer. Place them (they should still be wet) in a skillet and dry-roast them until they pop, emit a nutty fragrance, and can be crushed easily between the thumb and index fingers. Be careful not to burn them.

Place the seeds in the suribachi with the salt and grind them together until the seeds are half crushed and are all coated with salt. Make gentle circular motions using the grooves on the sides of the suribachi. When the gomashio cools, place it in an airtight glass or ceramic container. (If it is still warm, moisture will collect inside the container and can cause spoilage.) Sprinkle gomashio over grains and vegetables.

Sesame seeds are high in calcium, protein, iron, phosphorous, vitamin A, and niacin.

Wakame Powder

   1 strip kombu, 10″

Gently wipe the wakame with a clean cloth to remove any surface sand or dust. Place it in a 350°F. oven for 10 to 15 minutes, or until it is crisp but not burnt. (While the wakame is in the oven, it may still seem wet. To test, remove a small piece and let it cool for a minute or two.) Grind the wakame to a fine powder in a suribachi. Use as a condiment for grains and vegetables.

Variations: Kombu and dulse can also be roasted this way and ground into a powdered condiment.

Wakame-Sesame Condiment

   1 oz. wakame
   1 cup sesame seeds, washed and dry-roasted

Place wakame in a baking pan and bake at 350°F. approximately 10 minutes, or until crisp. Break the wakame into small pieces and grind in a suribachi along with the sesame seeds until it forms a powder. Kombu and dulse can also be used in this recipe.

Variations: Condiments can be made this way using: kombu and sesame seeds; dulse and sesame seeds; dulse and sunflower seeds; wakame, shiso, and sesame seeds; kombu and pumpkin seeds; and so on.

Shiso Leaf Powder

Dry-roast 1 cup shiso leaves in a skillet or in the oven at 350°F. until it dries out. Grind in a suribachi until it forms a powder. This can be combined with seeds, sea vegetable powder, or both.

Nori Condiment

10 sheets nori, broken or cut into small pieces
1 cup spring water
½ Tbsp. tamari soy sauce

Bring all the ingredients to a boil in a small covered pot, turn the flame to low, and slowly simmer for about 20 to 30 minutes, or until most of the liquid has boiled away, leaving a paste of nori.

Wakame, Rice Vinegar Condiment

1 cup wakame, soaked and sliced
2 Tbsps. brown rice vinegar
2 Tbsps. soaking water from wakame
2 Tbsps. tamari soy sauce

Cook as in *Nori Condiment* (above), adding water, rice vinegar, and tamari soy sauce in the beginning with the wakame.

Shio Kombu

8 long strips (about 12″) kombu
Enough liquid to cover (50% water and 50% tamari soy sauce)

Cut the kombu into 1-inch squares with scissors and soak them in water/tamari for 1 to 2 days. Place them into an uncovered pot, add enough water/tamari to cover, bring to a boil, immediately turn the flame to low, place a heat deflector underneath, and slowly simmer for several hours, until most of the liquid has evaporated. Since this is very strong, have only one or two pieces at a meal.

Grated Daikon Condiment
(This can be used to help balance a meal containing fish, tempura, or a heavy, rich dish.)

$\frac{1}{4}$ **cup grated daikon**
$\frac{1}{4}$ **tsp. tamari soy sauce**
Optional: **Small amount of fresh grated ginger**

Mix together and serve. Serves 1.

Scallion-Miso Condiment

2 bunches scallions
2 Tsps. miso
1 capful rice vinegar
Spring water

Separate scallion roots and greens. Blanch the roots 1 minute in a small amount of boiling water, and the greens for about 30 seconds. Dilute the miso with the rice vinegar and a small amount of boiling water. Simmer the miso mixture 2 to 3 minutes, cool slightly, and pour over the scallions, which have been placed on a serving dish.

Roasted Soybeans and Miso

1 cup roasted yellow or black soybeans
1 cup sliced celery
1 cup diced onion
1 cup sliced lotus root
$\frac{1}{2}$ **cup diced carrots**
$\frac{1}{4}$ **cup burdock, thinly sliced**
1 Tbsp. sesame oil
1 Tbsp. miso
$\frac{1}{2}$**–1 tsp. fresh, grated ginger for garnish**

Dry-roast the soybeans, then soak them in 1 cup of warm water for 10 minutes. Meanwhile, slice the vegetables. In a pot, warm the sesame oil and add the vegetables in layers, beginning with the celery, then the onion, lotus root, carrots, and burdock.

Strain the roasted soybeans from the soaking water and put them on top. Add the strained soaking water to the pot gently, being careful not to disturb the order of the layers. Dilute the miso in a half cup of water and place on top of the soybeans. Cover the pot and cook for 10 to 20 minutes. The carrots and burdock should become soft, but not too soft. When done, garnish with grated ginger, mix well, and serve.

13. Sauces, Dressings and Garnishes ▬

Sauces and Dressings:────────────────────────────

In general, it is best to use sauces and dressings sparingly. When properly prepared, most macrobiotic dishes are attractive and delicious enough to stand on their own. However, sauces and dressings can be a nice addition at times, particularly with more bland or lighter dishes, and for parties and special occasions. They can add appeal, like condiments, without covering up the taste and other qualities of the dish they accompany.

Kuzu Sauce

1–1½ cups soup or vegetable stock
1 Tbsp. kuzu dissolved in a small amount of water
Tamari soy sauce to taste
Optional: 2–3 pinches grated ginger

Bring dissolved kuzu and soup stock to a boil, lower the flame, and simmer and stir until the kuzu becomes transparent. Then add the tamari soy sauce and ginger. Serve over grains or vegetables.

Kuzu Sauce with Vegetables

½ carrot, cut into thin matchsticks
1 onion, thinly sliced
2 cups water or stock
2–2½ Tbsps. kuzu dissolved in a small amount of water
Tamari soy sauce to taste
Optional: a few pinches grated ginger, chopped scallions, or
   chopped parsley

Bring the stock to a boil. Add the vegetables and simmer until almost soft. Add diluted kuzu and stir until the liquid becomes transparent. Add tamari soy sauce, simmer a few minutes more, and mix in scallions, parsley, or ginger if desired, just before serving.

Onion Butter

Enough thinly sliced onions to fill a pot
½" water
1–2 pinches sea salt

Fill a heavy-bottomed pot with onions. Add salt, about ½ inch of water, and cover the pot. Very slowly, on a low flame, bring this to a boil. Then, turn the flame down even lower, place a flame deflector under the pot, and simmer for 6 to 10 hours, until the onions dissolve to a golden brown paste.

Umeboshi Dressing

2 umeboshi plums
¼–½ tsp. minced onion
½ tsp. sesame oil
½ cup spring water

Purée the umeboshi and onion in a suribachi. Heat the oil for about 1 minute and add it to the other ingredients. Add the water and mix well.

Sour Tofu Dressing

3 umeboshi plums
Spring water
1 cake tofu
¼ cup sliced scallions or chives, for garnish

Put the pitted umeboshi plums in a suribachi and puree to a smooth paste. Add the tofu and puree until smooth and creamy, adding a little spring water to moisten, if necessary. Garnish with sliced scallions or chives. A little tamari soy sauce may be added to this recipe.

Tofu Dressing with Miso

8 ozs. tofu
⅛ cup mugi miso
2 Tbsps. brown rice vinegar
¼ cup spring water
2 Tbsps. finely chopped onion
¼ cup chopped parsley

Blend the tofu in a suribachi and add the miso which has been puréed with the vinegar and water. Mix in the onion and parsley and let sit at least 30 minutes before serving.

Miso-Rice Vinegar Dressing

2 tsps. miso
½ cup spring water

154

2 tsps. brown rice vinegar

Purée the miso in a little water in a suribachi then place in a pot and simmer for 2 to 3 minutes. Add the vinegar and the rest of the water and blend.

Tamari-Vinegar Dressing

Optional: $1/4 - 1/2$ tsp. sesame oil
1 Tbsp. tamari soy sauce
4 Tbsps. brown rice vinegar
1 Tbsp. fresh, grated onion
$1/2$ cup spring water

If using oil, heat it for about 1 minute over a low heat. Puree all the ingredients together in a suribachi and serve.

Carrot Miso Sauce

4–6 carrots
1 stalk celery
2 onions
$1/2$ tsp. dark sesame oil
2 Tbsps. miso or to taste
Chopped scallions and/or celery leaves
Water
1 pinch sea salt

Slice carrots into thin slices. Pressure-cook with about an inch of water and a pinch of sea salt for 15 minutes. Puree in a food mill or suribachi.

Dice onions and celery. Heat oil in a large skillet and sauté onions until transparent. Add celery and continue to cook until celery is just tender. Add carrot puree and miso which has been dissolved in a small amount of water. Simmer for 3 to 5 minutes more. Add chopped scallion and celery leaf and serve hot over whole wheat spaghetti, elbows, or shells.

Variations: Cooked, chopped seitan can be added, as well as cooked, chopped tempeh.

Barley Malt Kuzu Sauce

1 cup water
$1/4$ cup barley malt (or to taste)
1 to 2 Tbsps. kuzu
1 pinch of sea salt

Dissolve the kuzu in a small amount of cold water. Mix water, kuzu, salt, and barley malt in a small sauce pan. Bring to a boil over medium heat while stirring constantly. Simmer for 5 minutes and serve.

Fruit and Kuzu Topping

1 cup apple juice
$\frac{1}{2}$ cup sliced fruit or berries
2 Tbsps. kuzu
1 pinch of sea salt

Bring apple juice, fruit, and sea salt to a boil. Simmer on a low heat until the fruit is well-cooked. Dissolve the kuzu in a small amount of cold water and add to sauce while stirring constantly. When liquid becomes transparent, simmer 2 to 3 minutes more and serve.

Variations: Dried fruit can be substituted for fresh, water can be used instead of juice. More kuzu can be added to make a thicker sauce.

Garnishes

Garnishes are not to be forgotten in daily cooking. On one hand, they can delicately enhance the colors and appearance of your meals; on the other, they can add considerable dynamics in the areas of taste, texture, and energetics.

For instance, take a simple bowl of miso soup. By itself, it is strengthening and delicious. If you garnish that same bowl of soup (more yang) with fresh chopped scallions (more yin), the change is almost magical. The soup now is not only strengthening, but sweeter and more energizing as well.

Another example is a bowl of soba (buckwheat) noodles with tamari broth. Soba is a more yang food (tamari broth can be more yang also). A dish like this eaten without an added garnish, may leave you feeling heavy and weighted down. If you add fresh, grated ginger or chopped scallions (both much more yin than soba), the whole dish becomes much more charged. Not only are the colors more appealing, the sharp, pungent taste and the light, quick energy of scallions, (or the warm, active energy of ginger), make the soba a lot more zippy and energizing.

Some of the garnishes you could use are:
Chopped scallions   Toasted nori, cut into thin strips

Chopped parsley
Chives
Chopped or grated onion
Grated ginger
A sprig of watercress
A celery leaf
Sliced or grated red
  radish
Sliced or grated daikon
Croutons

Toasted white or black sesame seeds
Toasted pumpkin or sunflower seeds
Toasted almonds or walnuts
Sea vegetable powder
Sautéed vegetables
A lemon wedge
Raw vegetables or fruits cut into
  decorative shapes: a carrot
  flower, a cucumber fan, etc.

Examples for using garnishes include:

a. A rich, nishime-style dish with chopped parsley mixed in after cooking.
b. Thick, black soybean soup with a carrot flower, a dab of ginger, and a celery leaf in each bowlful.
c. A large serving platter of plain greens or pressed salad with toasted seeds sprinkled over.
d. A broiled fish fillet with a lemon wedge and a sprig of parsley.
e Strawberry kanten with a few almond slivers on top.
f. Feel free to create your own combinations.

14. Desserts ━━━━━━━━━━━━━

Delicious desserts can be made using squash, sweet grains, or azuki beans as a base, rather than fruit or flour. The best sweeteners for health are:

1. Amazaké, a drink or a pudding made from fermented sweet rice and a starter called koji, also made from rice. It can be consumed as it is, or added to other dessert recipes.
2. Rice syrup
3. Barley malt syrup
4. Chestnuts
5. Mirin, a cooking wine made from sweet rice. It is used more in regular cooking than in desserts
6. Raisins and other dried fruits such as apples, peaches, pears, apricots, currants, and cherries
7. Fresh seasonal fruits, cooked
8. Apple juice and cider

Agar-agar and kuzu are natural thickeners which can be used in place of eggs, gelatin, and the like.

For more extensive recipes on cookies, cakes, muffins, and so on, refer to other macrobiotic cookbooks. Since this book deals mainly with the healing process, these less healthful types of desserts are not included.

Amazaké
(Also sold ready-made in some natural food stores.)

4 cups sweet brown rice
½ cup koji (sold in some natural food stores)
8 cups water

Soak the rice overnight and pressure-cook it for 30 minutes. When done, place it into a glass bowl and, as soon as it becomes cool enough to handle, mix in the koji, cover with a towel, and put it in a warm place. An oven with just the pilot light on, or the radiator, will do. Let this ferment for 4 to 8 hours. Mix it once in a while to help dissolve the koji. The fermentation is done when bubbles start to appear on the surface and when the mixture begins to taste sweet. It becomes sweeter and sweeter up to a certain point and then starts to turn sour. Catch it when it is sweet, place it back into a pot, bring it to a boil, add a pinch of salt, and turn it off as soon as it starts to bubble.

Amazaké can be used as it is or blended in a food mill. For a delicious drink, after blending, add a small amount of water and optional grated ginger, bring to a boil, and serve. Or, let it cool off to make a refreshing cold beverage.

To keep the amazaké for a longer time, simmer it over a low flame with a heat deflector underneath until it becomes slightly brown.

Basic Amazaké Pudding

>4 cups amazake drink
>6 Tbsps. kuzu, dissolved in a small amount of water
>2 pinches sea salt
>*Optional:* $\frac{1}{4}$ cup raisins

Place all ingredients into a pot, and bring to a boil while stirring constantly with a wooden spoon to avoid lumping and burning. Then simmer for about 3 minutes, pour into a serving plate, let it set, garnish, and serve. If it jelled properly, you will be áble to slice it into squares. Serves 8.

Chestnut Sweet Rice

>2 cups sweet rice
>$\frac{1}{2}$ cup dried chestnuts
>3 cups spring water
>2 pinches sea salt

Wash the chestnuts (sort out the discolored ones) and dry-roast them for about 5 minutes in a skillet over a medium-low flame. Stir with a wooden spoon, making sure that they do not burn. Put them in a pressure cooker with sweet rice and cook as in *Basic Brown Rice*. Serves 4 to 6.

Sweet Azuki Beans

>1 cup azuki beans
>1 cup chestnuts
>$\frac{1}{8}$ cup raisins (or $\frac{1}{2}$ cup rice syrup)
>5 cups water
>$\frac{1}{2}$ tsp. sea salt

Soak azuki beans and chestnuts for 6 to 8 hours or overnight. Place all the ingredients except salt into a pressure cooker and pressure-cook for 40 to 45 minutes. Let the pressure come down completely. Add salt, bring to a boil again, turn flame to low, and simmer for another 15 to 20 minutes. Or, you can simmer for a longer time, in which case it will become even sweeter.

Ohagi

- 2 cups sweet rice
- 2 cups chestnuts
- 7 cups spring water
- 4 pinches sea salt
- $\frac{1}{2}$ cup black sesame seeds
- 1 Tbsp. tamari soy sauce

Dry-roast the chestnuts and pressure-cook them in 5 cups of water and 2 pinches of sea salt for 45 to 50 minutes. When done, blend it into a puree with a food mill.

Wash and dry-roast the black sesame seeds until they start to pop and emit a nutty fragrance. Put them into a bowl and pour the tamari on them.

Meanwhile, pressure-cook the sweet rice in 3 cups of water and 2 pinches of sea salt for 40 to 45 minutes. When it is done, vigorously pound the rice with a wooden pestle until the grains are half broken (in 15 to 20 minutes). Wet your hands and form the rice into small balls.

Coat some of the balls in sesame seeds and tamari by rolling them in the seeds. Coat the other ones in the chestnut puree by molding the puree onto them. Place them onto serving plates, creating some kind of attractive decoration with the two dif-ferent kinds of balls and some garnish. Serves 4.

You can also coat them with either the *Sweet Azuki Beans* dish mentioned above, some dry-roasted, finely chopped walnuts mixed with tamari or a squash puree.

Squash Pudding

- 1 medium-sized buttercup squash (about $2\frac{1}{2}$–3 lbs.)
- 1 cup spring water
- 1 pinch sea salt
- $\frac{1}{4}$–$\frac{1}{2}$ cup barley malt
- 1 Tbsp. kuzu
- 1 cup chopped walnuts

Wash squash and remove skin and seeds. Cut squash into chunks and place in a pot with the water. Add a pinch of sea

salt, bring to a boil, reduce heat to medium-low, and cover.
Simmer until the squash is soft, about 20 minutes. Puree the
squash in a hand food mill until smooth.
Return the pureed squash to the pot and add the barley malt.
Simmer for about 5 minutes. Dilute the kuzu in a little water
and add it to the pureed squash, stirring constantly to avoid
lumping. Simmer for 2 to 3 minutes. Remove from the heat
and allow to cool slightly. Pour into serving dishes. Serves 4
to 6.

Blueberry Couscous Cake

2 cups couscous *Optional:* ½ cup toasted, chopped walnuts
1 quart apple juice
¼ tsp. sea salt
1 pint blueberries

Bring apple Juice and salt to a boil. Add couscous and simmer
for 1 minute. Add blueberries and cook for a few seconds more.
Remove pot from heat and let set for 1/2 hour. Stir every 5 to
10 minutes to distribute liquid. (Stir very gently as to not
break the blueberries.) After ½ hour, mix in chopped walnuts
and press into a Pyrex dish. Let set for another ½ hour before
slicing. Serves 8.

Variations: Any fruit can be used in place of blueberries.
Dried fruit can also be used, soaking it in the apple juice until
tender. Almonds or pumpkin seeds can be used in place of the
walnuts. Cake can also be pressed into a mold to set. A sauce
of fruit and kuzu can be made to frost the cake. (See chapter
on *Sauces and Dressings.*)

Sweet Kuzu

1 tsp. kuzu
1 Tbsp. rice syrup or barley malt syrup
1 cup water

Dissolve the kuzu in 2 teaspoons of cold water until it becomes
a liquid. Put this in a pot with remaining water and sweetener.
Stirring constantly with a wooden spoon, bring this mixture to
a boil, turn the flame to low, and simmer for 10 to 15 minutes.
Serve hot.

Strawberry Kanten

2 cups strawberries

4 cups apple juice (or 2 cups juice and 2 cups water)
$\frac{1}{8}$ tsp. sea salt
1 bar agar-agar or 6 Tbsps. agar-agar flakes
1 Tbsp. kuzu diluted in a little cold water

Bring the liquid, salt, agar-agar, and kuzu to a boil, turn the flame to low, simmer and keep stirring until the kuzu becomes transparent and the agar-agar dissolves completely. Add the strawberries. Pour into a serving dish or bowl which has been rinsed with cold water. This dish can be varied by using other dried or fresh fruits and/or nuts. Serves 8.

Variations: Kanten can be made with just apple juice. Other fruit may be used in addition to or instead of strawberries. Dried fruit may also be used, adding it at the beginning. Roasted nuts can also be added. Other juices from local fruits in season may be used instead of apple juice. Kuzu can be omitted (it makes a creamy gelatin).

Dried Fruit Compote

$\frac{1}{4}$ cup raisins or currants
$\frac{1}{2}$ cup dried apples
$\frac{1}{2}$ cup dried apricots
3 cups spring water
2 Tbsps. kuzu

Soak raisins or currants, apples, and apricots in water at least 30 minutes. Add a pinch of sea salt to the fruit and bring to a boil over medium heat. Cover and simmer 20 minutes. Dilute kuzu with a little cold water. Reduce heat to low and add the kuzu to the fruit. Stir constantly until thick, simmer for 2 to 3 minutes, and serve.

Applesauce

8 apples, cored
Water
2 pinches sea salt
Optional: 1 Tbsp. kuzu (For those with an overly yin condition.)

Cut apple into $1\frac{1}{2}$-inch slices and place in a pot. Add about 1 inch of water and the sea salt. Bring to a boil, and simmer over low heat until apples are soft. Puree in a food mill and serve.

Peach Pie

8 ripe peaches
⅛ tsp. sea salt
½ cup kuzu

Cut peaches in half and remove pits. Slice into 1-inch pieces. Grind kuzu and salt to a fine powder in a suribachi. Mix with peaches.

Crust:

4 cups whole wheat pastry flour
½ cup corn oil
2 Tbsps. barley malt
2 pinches sea salt
Cold water

Mix together the flour and salt. Add oil and quickly and gently mix until it forms small beads in the flour. Add barley malt and enough water to form a dough, mixing quickly and gently. (Do not over-mix, as it will make the crust tough. The less the better.)

Separate the dough into two balls, one slightly larger than the other (this is for the bottom crust). Dust a sheet of wax paper with flour and place the dough on it. Cover with another layer of waxed paper and roll out the larger piece of dough between the two sheets (quickly and gently).

When the dough is about ¼-inch thick, transfer it to a pie plate. Add peach filling and roll out the other piece of dough. Lay it on top of the pie, trimming and sealing the edges where the two crusts meet. Cut a few holes on the top crust to let steam escape while baking.

Bake at 350°F. for 45 minutes. Turn heat to 425°F. and cook for 15 minutes more. Wait until cool before slicing. (You can put a cookie sheet on the rack under the pie while it is cooking to catch any drippings.)

Mochi Pie Crust

(This is a much healthier alternative to regular pie crust but is only practical for open-faced pies.)

Cook and pound sweet rice as in the *Mochi* recipe, but then, instead of using it as mochi, oil a pie plate and press the mochi into it and shape it as a pie crust. Then bake as usual. This does not need to be prebaked before adding filling.

This crust makes the most delicious vegetable pies. Tofu, seitan, tempeh, or natto can also be added. (For vegetable pies, a small condiment of grated daikon with tamari soy sauce or grated ginger will make a nice complement. This is not necessary for sweetened or fruit pies.)

Squash Pie

1 large cubed and peeled buttercup squash
1 cup barley malt
$\frac{1}{4}$ tsp. sea salt
$\frac{1}{4}$ cup water
$\frac{1}{2}$ cup dry-roasted, chopped walnuts

Pressure-cook squash, barley malt, water, and salt. Puree in a food mill. Place in a pot and simmer for 10 minutes. If it is too thick, add some more water. If it is too thin, cook until it thickens. It should be pretty thick. (Kuzu can also be added to thicken it.) Place in a prebaked pie shell and sprinkle chopped walnuts on top. Bake at 350° to 365°F. for $\frac{1}{2}$ hour, or until the crust is golden brown.

For a crust, use a mochi crust or half of the pie crust recipe from the *Peach Pie* recipe. (Bake crust at 425°F. for 10 to 15 minutes, or until golden brown.)

Chestnuts, fresh fruits, and other vegetables (unsweetened) can also be used as filling. Try making an onion pie with sautéed onions.

15. Fish ━━━━━━━━━━━━━━━━━

Fish should be eaten as fresh as possible, preferably the same day it is caught, or at least the same day it is purchased. Choose more yin, slow-moving, soft white-meat fish such as sole, flounder, haddock, carp, and so on, as opposed to more active, red-meat varieties such as tuna, salmon, swordfish, and the like. Temporarily avoid shellfish such as clams, oysters, mussels, shrimp, lobster, and crab.

It may be best for some persons to avoid fish entirely, at least for several months, or until symptoms have improved.

Eat two or three times the regular amount of hard leafy greens when including fish in a meal to help balance its strong yang energies. Grated daikon with a few drops of tamari and a bit of grated ginger will help neutralize any possible toxic side-effects of the fish. A few drops of lemon is helpful and a slice of lemon is a beautiful garnish as well.

Clear Fish Soup

> 1–2 fillets of sole (or other white-meat fish)
> 1 cup wakame, soaked and cut into 1″ slices
> 1 bunch watercress, previously boiled for 1 second
> 3 shiitake mushrooms, soaked and sliced
> 5–6 cups kombu stock (add shiitake soaking water)
> Tamari soy sauce to taste

Bring wakame, shiitake, and kombu stock to a boil, turn the flame down, and simmer for a few minutes until the wakame and shiitake soften. Cut the fish into 1½- to 2-inch pieces, and add them to the soup with tamari to taste. Simmer for 1 to 2 minutes or until the fish turns white. Ladle the soup into individual serving bowls and garnish with the watercress. Serves 6 to 8.

Fish Soup

> 6 ozs. cod or other white-fish fillets
> 6″-piece kombu
> 1 onion or leek, thinly sliced
> 1 stalk celery, thinly sliced
> 1 carrot, thinly sliced
> 6 cups spring water
> 4–5 Tbsps. kuzu, dissolved in a little cold water
> Tamari soy sauce

Chopped parsley for garnish

Combine kombu and water, and simmer, uncovered, over medium heat 3 to 4 minutes. Remove kombu and cut into squares. Return the kombu to the pot along with the vegetables, and simmer until they are soft. Cut the fish into chunks and add to the soup along with the tamari soy sauce and kuzu. Stir and simmer 3 to 5 minutes until the soup thickens. Garnish with chopped parsley and serve.

Koi Koku (Carp Soup)

1 small carp (about 2 lbs.)
Equal volume of thinly shaved burdock and/or carrots
1 cup bancha tea twigs and leaves (already used to make tea)
Enough liquid to cover, $\frac{1}{3}$ bancha and $\frac{2}{3}$ water
Grated ginger
Miso to taste, puréed
Clean 100% cotton cheesecloth

Buy a fresh carp, preferably a live one and ask the fish seller to kill and carefully remove the gallbladder and the yellow bitter thyroid bone. Leave the rest of the fish intact.

At home, chop the whole fish (bones, head, fins included) into 1-inch pieces.

Make a sack out of the cheesecloth and put the used bancha tea twigs inside. This helps to soften the fish bones.

Place all the ingredients, including the sack of tea twigs, but not the miso, into a pressure cooker. Pressure-cook for 1½ to 2 hours. Bring down the pressure, take off the lid, add the ginger and miso to taste, simmer for 5 minutes, and serve. Garnish with chopped scallions. Serves 6 to 8.

Variations: Red snapper or fresh-water trout can be used if carp is not available. Carrot can be used with or in place of the burdock to make a sweeter, milder soup. If you are cooking for just 1 to 2 people, this recipe is a lot of soup.
Rather than using just a piece of the fish, it is better to use the whole fish, and then either freezing or give away the extra soup.

Baked Scrod with Miso

1 cup barley miso
1 cup white miso

2 Tbsps. saké
½ cup mirin
1½–2 lbs. scrod fillets
Grated daikon

Puree the miso, mirin, and saké together thoroughly in a suribachi. Spread half the marinade over the bottom of a shallow baking dish. Lay the fish fillets on top of the miso spread. Then spread the remaining marinade on top. Let sit for 4 to 5 hours. Remove the fish from the marinade. Put the marinated fish in a baking dish and bake in a preheated 475°F. oven for 15 to 20 minutes. Serve with grated daikon.

Broiled Marinated Haddock

1½ lbs. fresh haddock fillets
3 Tbsps. tamari soy sauce
2 Tbsps. mirin
Lemon wedges

Rinse fish and pat dry. Combine the tamari soy sauce and mirin in a baking dish, and place the fish in the marinade, turning to coat both sides. Let the fish remain in the marinade about 15 minutes per side, basting occasionally.

Preheat the broiler. Place the fish fillets on a lightly oiled baking sheet, and pour a little marinade over them. Broil the fish 3 to 5 minutes, turn, spoon on a little more marinade, and broil another 3 minutes, or until the fish is thoroughly cooked. Remove fish to a serving plate and garnish with lemon wedges.

Fish and Corn Chowder

1 lb. cod	1 strip kombu, 6″
3 cups fresh corn kernels	Miso or tamari soy sauce to taste
2 onions	Chopped scallion
2 turnips	*Optional:* grated ginger
1 qt. water	

Make a stock by bringing the water to a boil and simmering the kombu for 5 minutes. Remove the kombu and save for another use. Dry-sauté the onions until golden brown and add to the stock with turnips and corn. Simmer for 10 minutes, or until vegetables are very soft. Cut the cod into 1-inch pieces and add to soup. Continue to cook until the fish is done. Season with miso, simmer for 1 minute more (without boiling), and serve garnished with chopped scallion and grated ginger.

16. Beverages

It is best to drink only when thirsty. Most of us drink out of habit, whether we want to or not (as we often do with eating). If often or strongly thirsty, some of the dietary reasons may include:

1) Overconsumption of salt
2) Overconsumption of animal products
3) Overconsumption of dry, baked and/or flour products
4) Overconsumption of spices
5) Overconsumption of food in general
6) Not chewing enough
7) Lack of fresh, light dishes
8) Excess of sea vegetables

Good-quality water, such as spring or well water is the best to use. Avoid distilled or highly chemicalized tap water as much as possible.

It is also best to avoid iced or cold drinks (even water), as they can shock and paralyze the digestive system and harden fat accumulations in the body.

The beverages used on a daily basis do not contain caffeine, sugar, carbonation, artificial color, preservatives, stimulants, or alcohol (particularly the hard-liquor varieties). If following the general "standard diet," occasional small quantities of more yin, good-quality drinks, such as green tea, beer, saké, and mint teas can be consumed. However, if an individual is trying to reverse a particular condition, these items are best avoided.

The recipes in the *Special Needs* chapter are to be used only when really necessary, and only for a short period of time.

Bancha Twig Tea (Kukicha)
(For daily use, the "brown rice" of beverages.)

1–2 Tbsps. bancha twigs
1½ quarts of water

Twig tea generally comes pre-roasted. If not, dry-roast the whole package of twigs and leaves in a skillet for 3 to 4 minutes, stirring gently with a wooden spoon. Set aside the 1 to 2 tablespoons to be used, and store the rest, after cooling, in an airtight jar until needed.

Add twigs to cold water, bring them to a boil, reduce the flame to low, and simmer 10 to 15 minutes, depending on the strength desired. While pouring tea into individual cups, use a bamboo tea strainer (available in natural or Oriental food stores) to strain out the twigs. A regular metal strainer can be used as an alternative. The twigs may be reused several times until they lose their strength, but make fresh tea on a regular basis.

Kukicha contains no caffeine, artificial colorings, or dyes, and is not aromatic. It aids digestion and helps to settle an acidic stomach as it is alkaline in nature. (Most teas are acidic.)

Mugicha (Roasted Unhulled Barley Tea)
(Good for daily or regular use.)

> 2 Tbsps. mugicha (available in natural food stores)
> $1\frac{1}{2}$–2 quarts of water

Place the mugicha in cold water, bring it to a boil, reduce the flame to low, and simmer several minutes. Cooking time depends on the strength of tea desired.

Homemade Grain Teas
(Good for daily or regular use.)

To make grain tea, wash and dry-roast any grain, including rice, millet, oats, barley, and wheat, in a dry skillet. Use a wooden spoon to stir. Store what is not needed immediately in an airtight container, after cooling, for later use. Take 2 tablespoons for $1\frac{1}{2}$ to 2 quarts of water and boil and simmer as in bancha tea.

Sweet Vegetable Drink

> 1 cup diced cabbage
> 1 cup diced carrots
> 1 cup diced onions
> 1 qt. water
> 1 pinch sea salt

Bring water, salt, and vegetables to a boil. Reduce heat to low and simmer from 20 minutes (for more yang conditions) to 45 minutes (for more yin conditions). Strain juice if desired for a clear drink. (Make sure you use the leftover vegetables in cooking. They can be made into soup, added to breakfast cereal, or eaten as is.) This drink can be enjoyed hot or cool.

Variations: Other sweet vegetables can be used, like winter squash, parsnips, fresh corn, and so on.

Yannoh/Grain Coffee/Root Coffee
(For more "occasional use.")

> 4 tsp. yannoh
> 4 cups of water

Bring yannoh and 4 cups of cold water to a boil. Immediately reduce the flame (as it will boil over), and simmer for several minutes.

Yannoh is sold in natural food stores but may be difficult to find. (When buying grain coffee, make sure that it does not contain fruits or more yin vegetables such as beets.) Below is a recipe for homemade yannoh.

Yannoh (Homemade)

> 3 cups brown rice
> 2½ cups wheat berries
> 1½ cups azuki beans
> 2 cups chick-peas
> 1 cup chicory root

Wash each ingredient, then separately dry-roast each until a nutty fragrance is emitted. Then grind and mix.

When cool, store the Yannoh in an airtight jar. For variety, experiment with different proportions of grains, beans, vegetables (like burdock or dandelion root), and chicory. One hundred percent dandelion-root coffee can be delicious.

Azuki Bean Tea
(For occasional use, and as a medicinal drink.)

> 1 cup azuki beans
> 3–4 cups water
> 1 piece kombu

Place kombu in the bottom of a pan, then add azuki beans and water. Boil, reduce flame to low, and simmer until the water becomes a rich red. Azuki tea is helpful when the kidneys are tight. Have one cup a day for 3 days.

Kombu Tea
(For "occasional use.")

> 1 strip kombu, 6″
> 2 cups water

Boil the kombu and water until only 1 cup of liquid remains.

Mu Tea
(For "occasional use" only.)

1 teabag Mu tea (sold in natural food stores)
4 cups water

Boil, reduce flame, and simmer for 10 minutes. Mu tea is made of a combination of either 9 or 16 different herbs. The mixture was concocted by my teacher, George Ohsawa, the man who first introduced macrobiotic principles to the Western countries.

Umeboshi Tea
(For "occasional use.")

3–4 umeboshi plums
1½–2 quarts water
Optional: 1–2 shiso leaves

Separate the meat of the umeboshi from the pits and tear it into several pieces. Add the umeboshi meat and pits to the water and bring to a boil. Turn the flame to low and simmer for 20 to 30 minutes. When cooled, this is a delicious, refreshing summer drink. It helps reduce thirst and replaces minerals lost by excessive sweating.

Leftover Vegetable Juice
(For "occasional use.")

The leftover liquid from boiling or pressure-cooking vegetables makes a nice beverage. Just make sure that there is not a lot of concentrated salt in the water.

Vegetable and Fruit Juices
(For "occasional use.")

The juice of any "regular use" vegetable or seasonal fruit on the *Standard Dietary Suggestions* list may be taken once in a while. In the winter it is preferable to heat juice up, especially the yinner fruit juices. They may be helpful occasionally to help relax an overly tight condition.

17. Special Needs ━━━━━━━━━━━

There are a variety of natural home remedies which may be helpful during the recovery process. For information about the duration of their use and the specific conditions for which they are recommended, please consult the companion book in the *Macrobiotic Health Education Series* as well as *Macrobiotic Home Remedies*, both by Michio Kushi.

Internal Remedies: ━━━━━━━━━━━━━━━

Agar-agar with Rice Syrup or Barley Malt
(To relieve constipation.)

$1\frac{1}{2}$ Tbsps. agar-agar flakes
1 Tbsp. rice syrup or barley malt
1 cup spring water
1 pinch sea salt

Bring all the ingredients to a boil, turn the flame down, and simmer 5 to 10 minutes. Remove the pot from the stove and take this drink while it is still warm.

Daikon Tea

2 Tbsps. grated daikon
A few drops tamari soy sauce
1 teacup hot bancha tea

Place daikon and tamari soy sauce in a drinking cup, fill the cup with hot bancha tea, stir, and drink. This drink may be used once a day for 2 to 3 days.

Carrot-Daikon Tea

1 Tbsp. grated carrot
1 Tbsp. grated daikon
A few drops tamari soy sauce
1 teacup hot bancha tea

Place the grated carrot and daikon, and the tamari soy sauce in a drinking cup, fill the cup with hot bancha tea, stir, and drink. This drink may be taken once a day for three days.

Kombu Tea

2 cups spring water
1 piece kombu, 3"–6"

Bring kombu and water to a boil, reduce the flame to low, and simmer until only 1 cup of water remains. Drink this two to three times per week.

Tamari Bancha

A few drops tamari soy sauce
1 teacup hot bancha tea

Place of few drops of tamari soy sauce into a teacup. Pour in hot bancha tea, stir, and drink. Use this drink on occasion, as needed.

Ume-Sho-Kuzu

1 heaping tsp. kuzu
1 tsp. tamari soy sauce
1 umeboshi plum, seed removed
1/8 tsp. fresh, grated ginger
1 cup spring water

Chop the meat of the umeboshi plum and put it aside. Dissolve the kuzu in a teaspoon of water until it becomes a liquid, then add it to a small pot with 1 cup of water. Bring this to a boil, then turn the flame to low, and stir constantly with a wooden spoon. When the mixture becomes transparent, add the tamari soy sauce, umeboshi, and ginger. Drink hot.

Shredded Daikon Tea

1/4 cup shredded, dried daikon
2 cups water
1 pinch sea salt

Boil the shredded, dried daikon (available in many natural food stores) in 2 cups of water and the sea salt until only 1 cup remains. Drink hot.

Lotus Seeds and Kombu

1/2 cup lotus seeds soaked overnight
1 strip kombu, 3" soaked and cut into thin matchsticks
Tamari soy sauce
Enough water to cover seeds

Bring the lotus seeds, kombu, and water to a boil, then turn the flame to low and simmer about 30 minutes, until the seeds and kombu become soft. Then add a few drops of tamari soy sauce to taste and simmer another 5 minutes. You can also use fresh or dried lotus root.

External Treatments:

Ginger Compress
(Helps circulation, and softens and dissolves mucus, cysts, tumors, and the like.)

> **6 Tbsps. grated ginger**
> **1 gallon water**
> **Cheesecloth 6" by 6"**
> **Rubber gloves**
> **3 cotton towels**
> **Optional: hot plate**
> **(A person to give the treatment. It is awkward and not relaxing to do it on oneself.)**

Bring a pot of water to a boil and turn the flame off. Meanwhile, make a sack out of cheesecloth, place the grated ginger inside, and tie the open end into a knot to close it. Immediately after turning off the flame and the bubbles have disappeared, squeeze as much ginger liquid as possible out of the sack and into the pot of water. Then, place the whole bag inside. The point is to put the ginger in water as hot as possible without boiling it, as boiling would cancel its effectiveness.

Lay the person who will receive the ginger compress on a bed or some cushions and let him or her relax. Put on the rubber gloves. Holding on to the two ends of a cotton towel, dip as much of it as possible into the water. Wring it out, and place it on the area of the body to be treated. If it is too hot, shake the towel a bit before applying it. Ideally, the towel should be as hot as one can stand. Cover it with a dry cotton towel to keep it warm for a longer time. Place another towel in the water and when the first towel has cooled off, wring this one out and exchange it with the first. Again, cover with the dry towel. Continue alternating the towels until the area being treated becomes red. The water can be reheated (but not boiled) if it becomes too cool.

The ginger compress is a wonderfully effective home remedy. In addition, it is inexpensive, easy to apply, and has no harmful side effects. However, there are situations in which the ginger compress should be used only as a preliminary to another application, and there are situations where it should not be used at all. Please consult a qualified macrobiotic teacher for guidance. Also, the book, *Macrobiotic Home Remedies* (see bibliography), offers a thorough explanation of this and many other natural applications.

Buckwheat Plaster
(Draws out excess fluid from swollen areas.)

> Buckwheat flour
> Enough hot water to form a hard, stiff dough
> 5%–10% grated ginger
> Clean cotton linen

Precede the plaster with a 5-minute application of the ginger compress on the swollen area. Form a dough with the flour, hot water, and ginger, and place a ½-inch layer on the affected area. Cover and tie it on with a strip of linen. Replace the buckwheat every 4 hours. The swelling should go down after several applications or at the most after 2 to 3 days.

Lotus Root Plaster
(Draws out excess mucus, especially from the sinuses, lungs, and bronchi.)

> 75%–85% grated fresh lotus root
> 10%–15% pastry flour
> 5%–10% grated ginger
> Cotton linen

Mix these ingredients and spread them ½-inch thick onto a linen cloth. Apply the plaster directly to the skin on the area

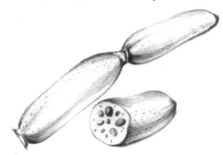

Fig. 21   Lotus Root

you are treating. Tie and keep this on for a few hours or overnight, and repeat this for a few days. It is helpful to do a ginger compress on the area before applying the plaster.

Daikon-Leaf Hip Bath
(For female sexual organ troubles.)

> 4–5 bunches dried daikon leaves (if unavailable, substitute 2 handfuls sea salt or 1 cup dried arame sea vegetable)
> 4–5 quarts water
> 1 handful sea salt
> A bathtub of waist-level hot water
> A towel

Dry several bunches of fresh daikon or turnip greens in the shade, until they become dry and brittle. (Dried daikon leaves can also be purchased in some natural food stores.)

Boil the dried tops with the handful of salt until the 4 to 5 quarts of water turns brown. Straining out the leaves, pour the liquid into the bathtub. The water in the tub should be hot and should come up to waist level. With a towel covering the upper part of the body, sit in the tub until the whole body becomes warm and begins to sweat (about 10 minutes). Do this for as many days as needed. Follow the bath with a bancha tea douche (see below).

Bancha Tea Douche
(For female sexual organ troubles.)

> Enough lukewarm bancha tea for douching
> $\frac{1}{2}$ tsp. sea salt
> Juice from half a lemon or equivalent amount of brown rice vinegar

Combine all the ingredients and use as a douche after taking the daikon leaf hip bath.

Greens with Bran Plaster
(Help to reduce discomfort from skin irritation or inflammation.)

> 50% rice bran
> 50% finely chopped, raw, green leafy vegetables
> A little water to help make a paste
> Cotton linen

Crush the hard, leafy, chopped greens (such as collards, kale, watercress, etc.) in a suribachi until they turn into a pulp. Combine with the bran and some water to make a paste. Apply the plaster on the feverish area and remove it when the paste becomes warm or hot.

Greens with Nori Plaster
(Helps to reduce discomfort from skin irritation or inflammation.)

Finely chopped raw, green leafy vegetables
A few sheets of nori

Crush the greens (such as collards, kale, watercress, etc.) and nori in a suribachi until they become a pulp. Apply this on the feverish area until the paste becomes warm or hot.

Tofu Plaster

1 cake fresh tofu
Equivalent amount of finely diced cabbage
Enough whole wheat flour to hold it together, about 10%–20% of the plaster.
1 tsp. grated ginger

Grind the tofu and cabbage into a paste in a suribachi. Add the ginger and flour, and place this mixture on a cheesecloth or cotton cloth, forming a sack with the tofu mixture inside. Put this on the forehead or any affected area, using the cheesecloth to tie it in place. When the mixture becomes warm, perhaps in 2 to 3 hours, exchange it for a fresh application.

Rice Bran Wash

Use two handfuls of rice bran (nuka). Make a sack out of a cotton cloth or cheesecloth (several layers thick), put in the bran and tie it tightly. Use this to scrub your body when you take a bath or shower. It can be used several times until it starts to spoil. This is also good for skin rashes.

Glossary

Agar-agar—A white gelatin made from sea vegetable, used for making *kanten*. You can get it in bars or flakes.

Ame—A natural grain honey derived from rice, barley, or wheat.

Amazake—A sweet porridge or drink made from fermented sweet rice. You can make this at home or buy it in some natural food stores.

Arame—A variety of sea vegetable.

Arepas—Corn cake made from *masa* corn dough.

Arrowroot—A finely ground white flour, used as a thickener, similar to *kuzu* and corn starch.

Azuki beans—Small, red beans. They are good for the kidneys.

Bancha—Tea made from a tea bush which is at least three years old. It helps digestion, and is good for daily use.

Burdock—A long, thin, dark, black root which grows all over the United States, as well as in other parts of the world. It gives one strength and stamina.

Couscous—A partially refined cracked wheat. It is light and cooks quickly. It is good for summer cooking.

Daikon—A long, thick, white root from the radish family. It is pungent when raw and is sweet when cooked. It is an excellent cleanser and purifier of blood, as it helps to break down fat deposits. Grated raw and served with a drop of *tamari* soy sauce, it is a good garnish with oily, greasy foods, making them more digestible.

Dulse—A variety of sea vegetable harvested in Maine, among other places.

Fu—Derived from wheat gluten, you can buy it in natural food stores in either flat, thin sheets, or in round donut shapes. When dry it is like a cracker but when cooked it is more like a noodle. A fun food.

Ginger—A hot, pungent, gnarly-looking, flesh-colored root. It adds zest to your dishes, and also helps circulation whether taken internally or applied externally as in a ginger compress.

Ginger compress—An external treatment made from grated ginger and hot water. It stimulates circulation, and unblocks stagnation (*see recipe*).

Gomashio—A condiment made from roasted sesame seeds and sea salt.

Hijiki—A black stringy variety of sea vegetable.

Hokkaido squash—A delicious squash, similar to buttercup.

Jinenjo—A very hardy, long, flesh-colored, mountain root potato. When grated it becomes a sticky mass and can be eaten with grains, or you can slice it and add it to vegetable dishes. It gives one strength.

Kanten—A gelatin-type food made from agar-agar. It makes a great light dessert when made with fruit and fruit juice. It is also used for aspics.

Kasha—Buckwheat groats.

Kinpira—A thinly sliced or shaved, sautéed-burdock dish, with or without carrots, and seasoned with *tamari* soy sauce.

Koji—Rice which has been innoculated with a form of bacteria. It is used as a starter for making *amazake, saké, miso,* and *tamari* soy sauce.

Kombu—A long, smooth, flat, thick variety of sea vegetable used in soup stocks, vegetable, bean, and grain dishes, and condiments.

Kukicha—Another name for *bancha*.

Kuzu—A starch made from the root of the *kuzu* plant (called *kudzu* in the United States), which is used as a thickener in vegetables dishes, and for medicinal purposes. When you buy it, it looks like little white rocks.

Lotus root—A tubular, flesh-colored root from the water lily family. It is hollowed out by several lengthwise airholes. It is good for the respiratory system and helps to unclog the sinuses.

Lotus seeds—Seeds of the above. They look like chick-peas.

Masa—A whole corn dough used as a base for *arepas, tortillas,* porridges, and so on. You make it at home but some natural food stores have started carrying it already made.

Mirin—A sweet wine made from rice and used in cooking.

Miso—A salty paste made from fermented soybeans with or without grains. Many varieties are available (see *Soups* chapter).

Mochi—Cakes made from pounded sweet rice which are dried and later used in a variety of dishes. It can be made at home or purchased in a natural food store. Make sure to get the brown rice variety instead of the white.

Mugicha—Tea made from roasted barley.

Natto—Stringy, fermented soybeans which when mixed with scallions, *tamari* soy sauce, grated ginger, and *daikon*, makes an excellent companion to a bowl of rice. The taste for it has to be acquired for some people. A good source of protein. It can be homemade or store bought.

Nishime—A method of cooking vegetables with a minimal amount of water.

Nori—A variety of sea vegetable which comes pressed into thin paperlike sheets. It can be used as a garnish, a cover for *sushi* and rice balls, and also as a condiment.

Norimaki—A type of *sushi* which is made by rolling *nori*, rice, and vegetables together into a long roll with a *sushi* mat.

Ohagi—Little balls of cooked, sweet rice which can be covered with seeds, nuts, or *azuki* beans, among other things.

Ojiya—A porridge of soft rice, vegetables, and *miso* (sea salt or *tamari* soy sauce can substituted for the *miso*).

Sea salt—Salt from the sea, much healthier than commercial land salt which contains iodine, sugar, and chemicals.

Seitan—Wheat gluten which has been boiled (and optionally deep-fried as well) with *tamari* soy sauce, *kombu*, and water. It is a good replacement for meat.

Shiitake—A variety of dried mushroom which is helpful in breaking down animal fats within the body. It is used as a soup stock or in vegetable dishes.

Shio kombu—A condiment made from *kombu* and *tamari* soy sauce.

Shiso—Beefsteak plant leaves which are pickled with *umeboshi* plums for added color. It strengthens blood quality, and can be used as a condiment.

Soba—Japanese buckwheat noodles.

Somen—An extremely thin variety of Japanese wheat noodles.

Suribachi—A ceramic bowl with grooves, used with a pestle for grinding and puréeing.

Sushi—Rice formed into little balls and topped with fish or vegetables, as well as rolls (*norimaki*) made from *nori*, rice, and vegetables.

Sushi mat—Bamboo mat used for making *norimaki sushi*.

Takuan—*Daikon* rice-bran pickles.

Tamari—A name given to naturally made soy sauce to differentiate it from the commercially made, chemicalized ones.

Tekka—A strong condiment made out of burdock, carrots, lotus root, ginger, *miso*, and sesame. Available in natural food stores.

Tempeh—Cakes of fermented soybeans, used widely in Indonesia, and available in natural food stores. A good source of protein.

Tofu—A white cake made from soybeans and water, also known as bean curd, available fresh or dried.

Udon—Japanese wheat noodles.

Umeboshi—Salty pickled plums. Helps cleanse the blood and aids digestion.

Wakame—A thin, leafy variety of sea vegetable.

Yannoh—Grain beverage sometimes used as a coffee substitute—made from five different grains.

Bibliography

Macrobiotic Health Education Series

Kushi, Michio. *A Natural Approach: Allergies*. Edited by Mark Mead and John D. Mann. Tokyo: Japan Publications, Inc., 1985.

————. *A Natural Approach: Arthritis*. Edited by Edward Esko and Charles Millman. Tokyo: Japan Publications, Inc., 1988.

————. *A Natural Approach: Diabetes and Hypoglycemia*. Edited by John D. Mann. Tokyo: Japan Publications, Inc., 1985.

————. *A Natural Approach: Infertility and Reproductive Disorders*. Edited by Charles Millman and Phillip Jannetta. Tokyo: Japan Publications, Inc., 1987.

————. *A Natural Approach: Obesity, Weight Loss and Eating Disorders*. Edited by John D. Mann. Tokyo: Japan Publications, Inc., 1987.

Macrobiotic Food and Cooking Series

Kushi, Aveline. *Cooking for Health: Allergies*. Edited by Rosalind Rhodes. Tokyo: Japan Publications, Inc., 1985.

————. *Cooking for Health: Arthritis*. Edited by Wendy Esko. Tokyo: Japan Publications, Inc., 1988.

————. *Cooking for Health: Diabetes and Hypoglycemia*. Edited by Rosalind Rhodes. Tokyo: Japan Publications, Inc., 1985.

————. *Cooking for Health: Infertility and Roproductive Disorders*. Edited by Helaine Honig. Tokyo: Iapan Publications, Inc., 1987.

————. *Cooking for Health: Obesity, Weight Loss and Eating Disorders*. Edited by Helaine Honig. Tokyo: Japan Publications, Inc., 1987.

Cookbooks

Aihara, Cornellia. *Macrobiotic Kitchen*. Tokyo: Japan Publications, Inc., 1983.

Esko, Edward and Wendy. *Macrobiotic Cooking for Everyone*. Tokyo: Japan Publications, Inc., 1980.

Esko, Wendy. *Introducing Macrobiotic Cooking*. Tokyo: Japan Publications, Inc., 1978.

Estella, Mary. *Natural Foods Cookbook: Vegetarian Dairy-free Cuisine*. Tokyo: Japan Publications, Inc., 1985.

Kushi, Aveline. *How to Cook with Miso*. Tokyo: Japan Publications, Inc., 1978.

Kushi, Aveline, with Alex Jack. *Aveline Kushi's Complete Guide to Macrobiotic Cooking for Health, Harmony, and Peace*. N. Y.: Warner Publishing Co., 1984.

Kushi, Aveline, with Wendy Esko. *The Changing Seasons Macrobiotic Cookbook*. Wayne, N. J.: Avery Publishing Group, 1984.

Ohsawa, Lima. *Macrobiotic Cuisine*. Tokyo: Japan Publications, Inc., 1984.

Other Macrobiotic or Related Books

Aihara, Herman. *Basic Macrobiotics*. Tokyo: Japan Publications, Inc., 1985.

Brown, Virginia, with Susan Stayman. *Macrobiotic Miracle: How a Vermont

182

Family Overcame Cancer. Tokyo: Japan Publications, Inc., 1985.

Dufty, William. Sugar Blues. New York: Warner, 1975.

Kohler, Jean and Mary Alice. Healing Miracles from Macrobiotics. West Nyack, N.Y.: Parker, 1979.

Kotzsch, Ronald E. Macrobiotics: Yesterday and Today. Tokyo: Japan Publications, Inc., 1985.

Kushi, Aveline. Lessons of Day and Night. Wayne, N. J.: Avery Publishing Group, 1984.

Kushi, Michio. The Book of Dō-In: Exercise for Physical and Spiritual Development. Tokyo: Japan Publications, Inc., 1979.

Kushi, Michio. The Book of Macrobiotics (Revised edition), Tokyo: Japan Publications, Inc., 1987.

———. Cancer and Heart Disease: The Macrobiotic Approach to Degenerative Disorders (Revised edition), Tokyo: Japan Publications, Inc., 1985.

———. The Era of Humanity. Edited by Sherman Goldman. Brookline, Mass.: East West Journal, 1980.

———. How to See Your Health: The Book of Oriental Diagnosis. Tokyo: Japan Publications, Inc., 1980.

———. Macrobiotic Home Remedies. Edited by Marc Van Cauwenberghe. Tokyo: Japan Publications, Inc., 1985.

———. Natural Healing through Macrobiotics. Tokyo: Japan Publications, Inc., 1987.

———. Your Face Never Lies. Wayne, N.J.: Avery Publishing Group, 1983.

Kushi, Michio and Aveline. Macrobiotic Pregnancy and Care of the Newborn. Tokyo: Japan Publications, Inc., 1984.

———. Macrobiotic Child Care & Family Health. Tokyo: Japan Publications, Inc., 1986.

Kushi, Michio, with Alex Jack. The Cancer Prevention Diet. N. Y.: St. Martin's Press, 1983.

———. Diet for a Strong Heart: Michio Kushi's Macrobiotic Dietary Guidelines for the Prevention of High Blood Pressure, Heart Attack, and Stroke. New York: St. Martin's Press, 1985.

Kushi, Michio and the East West Foundation. Cancer and Heart Disease: The Macrobiotic Approach to Degenerative Disorders. Edited by Edward Esko. Tokyo: Japan Publications, Inc., 1982.

Mendelsohn, Robert, S. Confessions of a Medical Heretic. Chicago: Contemporary Books, 1979.

———. Male Practice. Chicago: Contemporary Books, 1980.

Nussbaum, Elaine, Recovery: From Cancer to Health Through Macrobiotics. Tokyo: Japan Publications, Inc., 1985.

Ohsawa, George. Cancer and the Philosophy of the Far East. Oroville, Calif.: George Ohsawa Macrobiotic Foundation, 1971.

Ohsawa, George, with William, Dufty. You Are All Sanpaku. N. Y.: University Books, 1965.

Sattilaro, Anthony, with Tom Monte. Recalled by Life: The Story of My Recovery from Cancer. Boston: Houghton-Mifflin, 1982.

Tara, William. Macrobiotics and Human Behavior. Tokyo: Japan Publications, Inc., 1985.

Index

189